"The management of eating disorders presents unique challenges to health care professionals, families and sufferers. Having an eating disorder is not a choice and the consequences of these illnesses can be dire. Dr. Kirkpatrick's book *Medical Crises in Eating Disorders* uses clinical stories to help simplify and humanize these complex illnesses and serves as an excellent tool to better understand the medical needs of those affected and their families."

Dr. Julia Raudzus, *MD, FRCPC, Medical Director,*
BC Provincial Tertiary Adult Eating Disorders Program,
St. Paul's Hospital

"James R. Kirkpatrick speaks to the eating disorder clinician and encourages us to delve deeper into the myriad of behavioral, psychological, and medical symptoms of our patients. He emphasizes the precariousness of these life-threatening illnesses and the need for crisis prevention."

Esther J. Dechant, *MD, Medical Director,*
Klarman Eating Disorders Center, McLean Hospital and
Assistant Professor of Psychiatry, Harvard Medical School

Medical Crises in Eating Disorders

Medical Crises in Eating Disorders provides medical clinicians as well as others with an acute awareness of the critical and potentially lethal medical outcomes they may have to face when managing those with eating disorders.

This book shares multiple blended patient stories that cover a wide range of medical crises and present a realistic clinical-like experience. The reader will gain insight into the most threatening medical risks described in medical terms and many of the behaviors utilized by those with eating disorders that lead to most of the critical, including lethal, medical risks. Non-eating disorder causes of risk are also discussed throughout the book. Examples of electrocardiogram images, echocardiogram reports, and blood and urine results in addition to hospital chart vital records and excerpts from official coroner's documents help augment the learning experience.

This innovative book is a necessary reference for those who manage the medical concerns of those with eating disorders, including critical care physicians, internists, pediatricians, psychiatrists, and family physicians. As well, psychologists, counselors, dietitians, nurse practitioners, and social workers will benefit from an increased awareness of critical medical risks.

James R. Kirkpatrick, MD, has managed the care of adolescents and adults with eating disorders for more than thirty years. He has been a clinical assistant professor at the University of British Columbia, as well as a member of the Academy for Eating Disorders and the World Health Organization's Global Clinical Practice Network.

Medical Crises in Eating Disorders

James R. Kirkpatrick

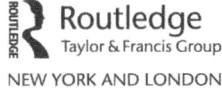
Routledge
Taylor & Francis Group

NEW YORK AND LONDON

Cover image: provided and owned by the author

First published 2023
by Routledge
605 Third Avenue, New York, NY 10158

and by Routledge
4 Park Square, Milton Park, Abingdon, Oxon, OX14 4RN

Routledge is an imprint of the Taylor & Francis Group, an informa business

Library of Congress Cataloguing-in-Publication Data
Names: Kirkpatrick, Jim, Dr., author.
Title: Medical crises in eating disorders / James R Kirkpatrick.
Description: New York, NY : Routledge, 2023. | Includes bibliographical references and index. |
Identifiers: LCCN 2022016779 (print) | LCCN 2022016780 (ebook) | ISBN 9780367512651 (hardback) | ISBN 9780367512644 (paperback) | ISBN 9781003053088 (ebook)
Subjects: LCSH: Eating disorders. | Eating disorders--Treatment.
Classification: LCC RC552.E18 K556 2023 (print) | LCC RC552.E18 (ebook) | DDC 616.85/26--dc23/eng/20220628
LC record available at https://lccn.loc.gov/2022016779
LC ebook record available at https://lccn.loc.gov/2022016780

ISBN: 978-0-367-51265-1 (hbk)
ISBN: 978-0-367-51264-4 (pbk)
ISBN: 978-1-003-05308-8 (ebk)

DOI: 10.4324/9781003053088

Typeset in Baskerville
by MPS Limited, Dehradun

For Stew, Margaret, Ian and Sara just for being there.

Contents

About the Author

James R. Kirkpatrick is a founding member of the B. C. Eating Disorders Association. He has been a medical consultant for the Ministry of Health as well as the South Vancouver Island Eating Disorders Program of the Ministry of Children and Family Development in Victoria, British Columbia, for almost three decades. He completed his undergraduate education as well as medical training from the Department of Family Medicine, Faculty of Medicine at the University of Saskatchewan. He is editor emeritus for the journal *Eating Disorders: The Journal of Treatment and Prevention*. Dr. Kirkpatrick is a retired clinical assistant professor for the Department of Psychiatry, Faculty of Medicine, University of British Columbia and the Island Medical Program at the University of Victoria. He has been a member of the World Health Organization's Global Clinical Practice Network and the Academy for Eating Disorders. As well as his work in the field of eating disorders, he has been a clinician at the Island Sexual Health Society for twenty-seven years. The Canadian Medical Association commissioned his book, *Eating Disorders* (Kirkpatrick & Caldwell). He was honored with the B.C. Community Achievement Award by the lieutenant governor of British Columbia in 2015 for advocacy and leadership in developing treatment for those with eating disorders, university teaching and clinical dedication. Dr. Kirkpatrick has been a civilian Medical Officer for the Royal Canadian Navy and medical director for the Victoria Methadone Clinic. He has also published a music instruction book, *Electric Bass Beginnings* and coauthored several neuroscience research papers. He currently resides in Victoria, British Columbia, with his wife, Gail, and has two children, Amy and Paul.

Preface

These are the last three cardiac tracings for Angel. She was someone with severe anorexia nervosa who said she vomited 20 times during each of 4 sessions of vomiting daily. That is, she was vomiting about 80 times a day. She experienced chronic metabolic alkalosis as well as hypomagnesemia and had been admitted to the coronary ICU two months earlier with a torsades de pointes cardiac rhythmic pattern observed while wearing a Holter monitor – a dysrhythmia that can be a precursor to sudden cardiac death. Below are sequential tracings taken seconds apart during a failed resuscitation attempt by paramedics in her home. (Figures 0.1, 0.2, and 0.3.)

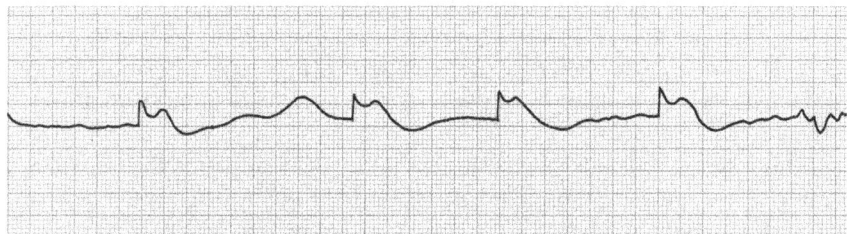

Figure 0.1 Agonal junctional rhythm.

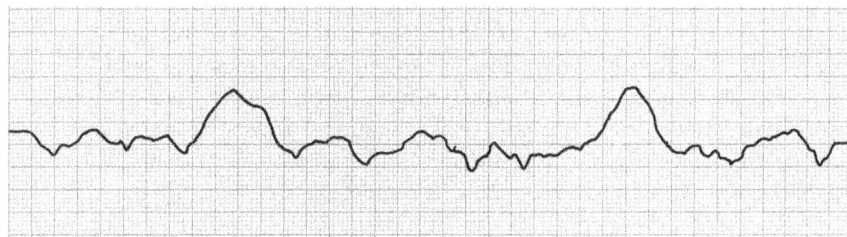

Figure 0.2 Polymorphic ventricular arrythmia.

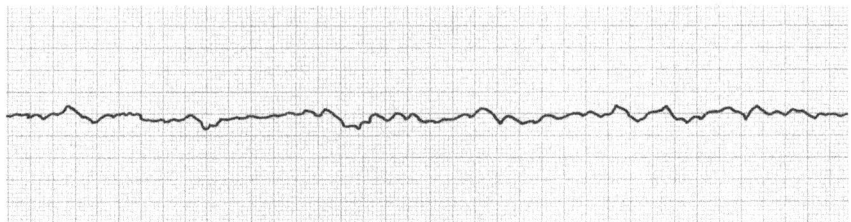

Figure 0.3 Fine ventricular fibrillation.

The coroner's report states "There were bags of prescription magnesium and potassium supplements in her bedroom." *From her history and these tracings she likely died from sudden cardiac death.*

Angel's story defines the purpose of this book, *Medical Crises in Eating Disorders*. Trying to prevent similar outcomes as Angel's in high-risk individuals with eating disorders is its ultimate goal – a task of immeasurable importance. For clinicians, the book highlights many of the terrorizing medical and psychological risks that keep us awake staring at the ceiling at three in the morning as we wonder if we have done enough. Have we put individuals at risk by our actions or lack of actions? Did we zig when we should have zagged?

The best way to preempt crisis is by being aware, ahead of time, factors that create crisis or allow crisis to evolve unchecked. As well, we need to know how to deal with a crisis should it occur. There is little point in anticipating a potential crisis if we don't have the resources to manage it or are not present when a crisis happens.

This is not a book advising treatment for medical or psychological issues. It provides awareness of those medical crises that may be around the corner or of a crisis already in the making that we may not be able to see when it is right before us.

No Warning ... Usually

The majority of health issues that become critical often have an observable evolution of symptoms and signs. We might be able to say "I could see that coming." Individuals with a kidney infection will usually have symptoms of flank pain, dysuria, and likely fever. As the infection becomes more aggressive the person feels sicker and weaker and others can observe the illness progressing. A medical crisis such as meningitis that can hit hard and fast creating symptoms such as severe head pain, fever, and a profound sense of feeling unwell can be noticed by family and clinicians as it progresses. In these instances there would often be enough time to make an accurate diagnosis and provide appropriate treatment. With medical crises in those with eating disorders there are often *no warning signs or symptoms prior to demise.*

Typical real-life stories of those with eating disorders include a young woman dropping dead while playing tennis, teaching a high school class, or watching television. Individuals may die of sudden cardiac death while driving through a busy intersection. All of the above individuals had been engaged in active daily functions as if there was nothing seriously wrong with their health. None had been lying in an ICU hospital bed hooked up to life-support technology with highly skilled medical caregivers at their bedside or in a hospice facility as would be the case for those with other terminal illnesses. Those with eating disorders just "drop dead" midstride. No warning. Almost no one with an eating disorder dies in the hospital from medical causes. They typically die of eating disorder related causes in the community. They may also die of non-eating disorder specific health issues in the community especially if not being closely monitored such as those with insulin-dependent diabetes mellitius or at risk of suicide.

Aside from direct medical crises, suicide deaths also usually occur without warning. We are typically, however, surprised when it does happen at one given moment in time. Medical personnel need to understand that we are just as responsible for suicidal deaths as other clinicians. We must be just as aware of warning signs, if any, and be as prepared to deal with them as best we can. For some of those with chronic and severe eating disorders, we are often surprised that death from direct medical causes or suicide hasn't happened earlier.

All Suicides are Medical Deaths

Though no surprise to anyone, all deaths by suicide are the result of medical demise. Individuals either die of cardiac or respiratory compromise – the same as all those that die from metabolic instability, renal failure, or congenital cardiac anomalies. As clinicians we tend to think of the care of those with eating disorders as either psychological or medical management – the medical people take care of the medical concerns and the counselors or therapists take care of the psychological issues including suicidal risk. Medical clinicians need to look upon suicidal risk in the same light and importance as pure medical risks.

Statistics

Statistics have been provided where possible. However, reliable statistics are very limited overall as so much about eating disorders have not been researched adequately. Much of the statistics available in the literature is dated and for various reasons inaccurate. A lack of statistical analysis regarding medical crises risk does not diminish their posing threats.

Eating Disorders Are Conditions of Extremes

While dealing with one set of extremes may be difficult enough, often there are multiple sets of extremes stacked on top of each other confounding life further.

Extremes of Body Image Dissatisfaction and Control

While many in society likely have some dissatisfaction with aspects of their body image, including weight, size, and shape, most will not go to great lengths to cope with this.

For those with eating disorders, extremes of body image distortion, self-loathing, contempt, and worthlessness prevail and individuals often go to extremes to correct their dislikes using a myriad of eating disorder behaviors.

Extreme Physical Goals

While some will want to lose 10–20 lbs in order to meet their weight loss goal, others may wish to lose 50–75 lbs and even more. I met a person with bulimia who lost 150 lbs. Another individual, a 25 year old adult woman with anorexia nervosa, weighed 26 kg or 57 lbs with a height of 5'3". While a BMI of 17.5 or lower is required to meet the weight criteria for anorexia nervosa, some attain a BMI of 11 and lower.

Some try to acquire a skeletal or concentration camp-like body where creating observable bony prominences and an emaciated body are the goals. Others may set goals of obtaining life-threatening dysrhythmias, falling, losing consciousness and, not too infrequently, death. Vomiting blood or experiencing chest pain may be the end point on a given day for some.

Extremes of Eating Disorder Behaviors

Extreme goals of body shape (cachexia) and weight loss may be decided upon. These goals are often desperately expected to be achieved through utilizing any number of eating disorder behaviors. With well over a hundred eating disorder behaviors accessible to control body image, there is a cornucopia of potentially destructive opportunities to carry out body size and shape control expectations.

Not only is there a seemingly endless set of eating disorder behaviors to chose from that, when used in combination, escalate risk significantly, but each behavior individually can be used to extreme elevating risk even further. As an example, some may chose to vomit infrequently in order to control body image while others may end up vomiting 30, 40, 50 times a day or more. The use of 50 or one-hundred laxative tablets a day may be the choice of others. Some may choose to engage 20, 30 or more individual eating disorder behaviors simultaneously creating a large arsenal of weight control options. With each given eating disorder behavior there may be several parameters or variables that direct its course, complicating the picture further.

Extremes of Medical Risks

Akin to *Extreme Physical Goals* above, risks of developing renal failure, lethal dysrhythmias, severe osteoporosis, brain damage as well as sudden death become a threat.

Extremes of Social Incapacitation

Those with eating disorders may experience extremes of social isolation as well as a lack of capacity to pursue academic, job, or career opportunities. Relationships with family, partners, friends, peers, or coworkers may decay.

Extremes of Mental Health Decline

For those with eating disorders who are already prone to depression, anxiety or psychosis, these symptoms may become severe and unmanageable. Escalation of eating disorder behaviors, drug and alcohol use as well a self-harm including suicidal acts may occur.

For those that have experienced emotional, physical or sexual abuse, feelings of guilt, shame, as well as worthlessness may become overwhelming and the eating disorder, drug and alcohol use or self-harm may be ways of coping.

Extremes of Financial Stress

Treatment for eating disorders can be very costly. For individuals and families that have good health insurance options, financial costs may not be a significant factor. However, for far too many, healthcare costs are not covered adequately or even at all. Accumulated bills of tens of thousands and possibly hundreds of thousands of dollars become a reality. As an example, some families sell their homes to cover, as an example, $700,000 medical bills especially for residential or hospital care. A heartbreaking resulting aftermath of all this treatment and expense can be that the one with the eating disorder, who may have demonstrated excellent nutrition and resulting weight gain during treatment, returns to their original anorexia nervosa weight and medical status.

Extremes of Resistance to Care

Most of us in society, when faced with a serious health issue, will seek medical, psychological, and other healthcare resources. For those with eating disorders, there is often a profound resistance to seeking or accepting help – from anyone. This includes family, friends, partners, dietitians, therapists, social workers, medical doctors, and others. This resistance to care is an important contributor to escalated health risks.

About This Book

There are four chapters, each of which, highlight specific topics of focus.

1. Introduction: While the *Preface* sets the tone of the book, that is, one of crisis awareness and the need for clinicians to be super diligent, *Introduction* expands on this theme. Here, the urgent reasons to anticipate and deal with crises when they occur is driven home. As important, are clear descriptions of how these crises occur without warning and we end up saying to ourselves "How could this have happened?" In-depth details itemize preventive measures to help identify crises before they happen and help to decrease risks. The possibility of a crisis, including lethal ones, presenting right in front of clinicians is made salient. Being prepared to deal with crises in an instant is paramount.

This chapter describes what is a crisis and what may not be. No physical signs or symptoms are too small that they can be ignored. The smallest or infrequent medical complaint or finding may be the harbinger for a very serious and even lethal outcome. Where minimal symptoms in a healthy individual experiencing infrequent palpitations may be minimally investigated unless escalating, in those with eating disorders a full-on thorough investigation is warranted right away. Infrequent fluttering in the chest in one with an eating disorder could be caused by ventricular fibrillation or torsades de pointe both of which are precursors to sudden cardiac death. Anorectics have been described as "the walking dead."

2. Stories of Critical and Lethal Medical Scenarios: *Stories of Critical and Lethal Medical Scenarios* become the primary vehicle in revealing critical medical challenges. Each case or story offers essential pieces of the medial puzzle clinicians may be faced to manage in real-life situations.

A number of stories end with the death of an individual. Others display potentially lethal outcomes if not dealt with expediently. Some stories describe a "hint" of risk for which we must be diligent in observing as these risks could end in catastrophe. Medical investigation reports help to bring a sense of clinical reality. Multiple dysrhythmias, severe metabolic abnormalities, cardiac anomalies, and sudden death including sudden cardiac death are only a few of the medical situations illuminated in these cases. Death as a result of someone being incorrectly diagnosed with an eating disorder is highlighted. Suicide is touched on as well.

For some stories, a coroner has created a report gleaned out of medical reports including those from the emergency room, verbal accounts from family and professional caregivers as well as autopsy findings. Excerpts from these reports have been presented. Each report ends in a summary or conclusion as to the factors that led up to death. Sometimes there are not enough facts to make definitive conclusions. These reports provide an aerial view of the evolution of events sometimes connecting the dots that could have predicted, to some degree, the lethal outcome that may have been preventable.

3. Critical Medical Conditions: *Critical Medical Conditions* delves into the most feared and destructive sources of medical risk. As the majority of critical medical conditions have been presented in *Chapter 2: Stories of Critical and Lethal Medical Scenarios* as well as *Chapter 4: Eating Disorder Behaviors*, only selected topics have been addressed here.

The *Cardiovascular Effects of Eating Disorders* includes a focus on cardiac and other cardiovascular risks including prolonged QT interval, myocarditis, cardiomyopathy, pericarditis, cardiac anomalies, valvular disease, and septal defects. Mitral valve prolapse with associated anatomical and functional cardiac changes as well as lethal dysrhythmias are included.

Sudden Death covers causes of sudden death in those with eating disorders from cardiovascular origins, hypoglycemia, asphyxia, gastric dilatation, gastric rupture, emetic use and sepsis.

Refeeding Syndrome highlights the serious and possible lethal risks of feeding individuals who have been chronically starved and who may also have associated electrolyte and mineral deficiencies, metabolic abnormalities as well as multisystem failure. The *Minnesota Starvation Experiment* opens a window into the physiological and, in particular, the psychological impact of chronic starvation.

Insulin Dependent Diabetes Mellitus and its effect on those with eating disorders is touched on as a most life-threatening condition.

4.   Eating Disorder Behaviors: This chapter describes in some detail the plethora of behaviors used by those with eating disorders that aid in controlling weight, body shape, and emotions. Medical risks associated with many of these behaviors have been highlighted. Familiarity with these behaviors is essential for clinicians attempting to anticipate and manage critical medical situations. The primary eating disorder behavior categories are:

- Purging Behaviors
- Calorie Burning and Metabolism Altering Behaviors
- Body Gauging Behaviors
- Binge Eating and Related Behaviors
- Restricting Eating Behaviors
- False Information
- Organizing Behaviors
- Symptom Management Behaviors
- Surgery and Other Cosmetic Altering Methods
- Substance Use

For brevity, some of these topics have been only touched on.

About Myself

My post medical training is in family medicine. Because there were no dedicated resources locally and little province wide, I was put in the position to deal with multiple aspects of care for those with eating disorders. Initially, I saw those with eating disorders in my private office in order to do medical monitoring but very quickly was required to manage eating disorder attitudes and behaviors. I dealt with urgent mental health concerns such as depression, anxiety, and suicidal ideation. I managed both eating disorder related health issues and typical family doctor medical situations. For a number of years, I also provided the maternity care of those with eating disorders. I spent many hours in delivery rooms.

It was necessary to provide both nutritional support and counseling for eating disorder and mental health concerns where possible. Curious about how those I saw on first consultation had heard about me, when I asked one woman she said she had seen my name and office phone number written on a woman's restroom stall at the university – a lofty recommendation to be sure.

Through my office practice, I admitted adolescents to pediatric wards and adults to any adult ward that had an empty bed, whether it be surgery, internal medicine, gastroenterology, and gynecology services. I also admitted to the emergency rooms in two hospitals as well as to the pediatric and adult psychiatric wards. I provided over 80,000 hours of call for emergency rooms and hospital wards during a twelve year period. I was very busy. Fortunately, I had a small cadre of specialists and nutritionists with whom I shared care. I gained a broad knowledge and experiential base from which this book has been derived.

As well as my eating disorder clinical work, I continued in general practice for some time. I also worked in a sexual health clinic for almost three decades. For a time, I treated those with drug addiction at a methadone clinic and was civilian Medical Officer with the Royal Canadian Navy. These various clinical engagements helped expand my base of knowledge for those with eating disorders.

Prior to becoming a physician, I was a touring and studio musician. My first published book was an instructional book for electric bass guitar. I play electric bass guitar, flute, and now classical guitar. My experiences of being tutored in music and collaborating with other musicians have provided me with a reservoir of artistic spirit that, in turn, helped me engage with those with eating disorders who have artistic muses. These experiences also assisted me in connecting with individuals who demonstrate other competitive aspirations such as those who strive to be elite athletes or entertain other muses. Having been a music teacher may also have helped me to communicate the abstract concepts that music and, indeed, eating disorders possess.

The world of eating disorders presents many challenges for clinicians. They may be very difficult, time consuming, and sometimes heartbreaking. Your dedication to work with those with eating disorders provides a humanitarian gift that few others are able or willing to offer.

James R. Kirkpatrick

Acknowledgments

Over the years I have had the wonderful privilege of being a part of the care of those with eating disorders and their families. I am also fortunate to have been able to work with so many dedicated and caring clinicians from various disciplines. I especially wish to thank my friend and colleague, Stephanie Ustina, for our association over the last three decades.

Thanks to Don Wilkes, Dr. Michael Brook, Dr. Alan Buckley, and the Mayo Clinic in Rochester, Minnesota for their part. Special thanks to Dr. Markus Sikkel for assisting with EKG interpretations. I greatly appreciate Kurt McBurney for giving me a tutorial in cardiac anatomy at the Island Medical Program's gross anatomy lab. The University of Victoria and the University of British Columbia very kindly provided access to their resources. Thanks to the Coroners Service of British Columbia, College of Physicians and Surgeons of B.C. and the Canadian Medical Protective Association for their guidance. Heather McKenzie, our community owes you an ocean of gratitude and may you finally be at peace.

I especially wish to thank my brother, Stew Kirkpatrick, for performing his digital graphic art magic on the cover image. Much appreciated.

I very much wish to thank Amanda Savageand Katya Porter of the editorial team at Routledge for their patience and for holding my hand through this project.

I lovingly wish to profusely thank my wife, Gail, and children, Paul and Amy, for their support over the years.

Chapter 1

Introduction

Mary's Story

Mary, a twelve-year-old girl, was admitted to the children's hospital with concerns regarding precipitous weight loss, refusal to eat as well as persistent nausea. She would vomit if she had been encouraged to eat. She soon died after admission.

At autopsy, she was diagnosed with Addison's disease, a wasting condition that may present with nausea, vomiting, and weight loss.

Discussion

Much of what I have to say about Mary is speculation as her story had been presented anecdotally at a conference. It does, however, open up a variety of possible scenarios we all need to consider before making a diagnosis and implementing treatment.

The most salient feature of this story is that the presenting symptoms for Addison's disease are virtually identical to what may present in someone who has an eating disorder. Mary had not been diagnosed and treated by the hospital's eating disorder team but by staff on a general pediatric ward. What went wrong?

One possibility is that Mary presented with symptoms just at the time when eating disorders had hit the ground running worldwide. The media was identifying celebrities with profound eating disorders, especially anorexia nervosa, and turning them into cultural icons. Movie, television, and pop music stars as well as elite fashion models with eating disorders came front and center. I remember hanging around A & M Recording studios in Los Angeles during the early seventies. I bumped into Richard Carpenter there of the music duo, *The Carpenters*. At that time no one could predict that his sister, Karen Carpenter, would be the poster woman for anorexia nervosa and become just as famous for her eating disorder as she was for her music. Karen did die ultimately from complications of anorexia nervosa.

DOI: 10.4324/9781003053088-1

Average women in society became themselves superstars when presented on talk shows with extremes of anorexia nervosa donning concentration camp style bodies. These women's achievements of weight loss became more coveted than being a celebrity. Television talk show hosts were dangling these emaciated, near death and, indeed, dying individuals in front of the public as examples of a horribly destructive illness so as to shock the public into fearing eating disorders. The result instead came across as free advertising for the most coveted desire by many in society – an easily accessible, effective and extreme weight loss set of behaviors. Instead of successfully informing the public of these devastating conditions, they educated a generation of largely girls and young women as to how to lose weight better. Much better. I met over a dozen young teen girls who adopted eating disorder behaviors just from watching talk shows. The goal post had been moved for dieting from "watching what you eat" and "cutting out sweets and exercising more" to eating 2 crackers a day, vomiting 10, 20, and 30 times or more a day. Weight loss goals went from wanting to lose 5–10 lbs and toning-up to losing 30, 40, or 50 lbs or more. Emaciated and bony became the new black in body image desire – not just thin. Excessive exercise, laxatives, appetite suppressants, metabolism boosters as well as diuretics were in the mix. A new level of self-loathing evolved resulting in extremes of self-harm including suicide.

Mary's demise could have resulted from how her admitting medical history was addressed and paid attention to. It is easy to understand how the diagnosis of anorexia nervosa could have been made initially. This is a twelve-year-old girl who presented, during the height of a media-driven eating disorder frenzy, with severe precipitous weight loss, nausea and vomiting, and refusal to eat. Either a history focused on "why" she was vomiting and refusing to eat had not been fully explored or her comments were ignored. If she had been asked how she saw her body image, her concerns regarding weight, and whether she had been trying to lose weight, a different conclusion as to the etiology of her symptoms may have been made. If she had responded to this line of questioning with "I am not trying to lose weight and I can't help vomiting if I eat because of nausea." Red lights should have gone on that this may not be of eating disorder origin. A possibility is that these kinds of comments had been made but ignored as it could have been assumed that she was lying to protect her weight loss drives. It used to be not infrequently that colleagues would say "She's just saying she isn't dieting or vomiting because anorexics lie all the time."

Another scenario here is that Mary could have had an eating disorder as well as Addison's disease. We need to remember that eating disorders can coexist with any other medical condition. Do not ignore one diagnostic possibility in favor of another, should both be correct, until a thorough history and medical investigations have proven one way or another.

Clinicians as well as the public were swayed by the eating disorder tsunami. Although we as professional caregivers feel we are objective, we too tend to be influenced by the media. Because Mary's symptoms looked immediately like anorexia nervosa, other causes of her symptoms were likely overlooked and not investigated. I remember when other health conditions were newly made public by the media such as narcolepsy, false memory syndrome, Asperger's syndrome, as well as attention deficit hyperactivity disorder. I am sure that the diagnoses of these conditions went up significantly after being given media attention with the likelihood of false diagnoses in the mix. There is a "Looks like a duck, swims like a duck, quacks like a duck, then it probably is a duck" mentality in our society. The problem with this is that in health care, many disorders look alike until properly scrutinized.

It's too easy to make a snap diagnosis based upon early presenting symptoms and signs. Creating *differential diagnoses* before making a definitive diagnosis is critical in our work. An immaculate, detailed eating disorder and medical history is paramount for *every* individual regardless of our level of familiarity and expertise in the eating disorder field. Generalizations are dangerous as there are too many permutations and combinations of eating disorder behaviors and medical risks to be casual with our assessments.

As reinforced a number of times in this book, all symptoms that present in those with eating disorders may be associated with other health conditions either physical, mental, or a combination of both. The medical consequences of eating disorders may aggravate an existing non-eating disorder medical condition. As an example, a congenital dysrhythmia may be made worse by an eating disorder generated metabolic abnormality. Preexisting mitral valve prolapse may be worsened by eating disorder caused weight loss.

Crisis is in the Mind of the Beholder ..... Sort Of

There are overt medical and psychological crises. Cardiac arrest or suicide attempts are undisputable crises. What is not so obvious or as attention grabbing is when individuals themselves feel in crisis over what others might feel is not that important. We need to pay attention when someone says "I can't stand how fat I feel," or is upset because they have acne. Those who feel fat or otherwise hate their body can and do suicide. Someone with acne can absolutely hate themselves to the point of suicidal ideation including attempts. As with seemingly minor medical symptoms, we need to have a high index of suspicion for seemingly minor expressions of emotional discontent.

The concept of crisis is, to some degree, open to interpretation in some situations. This is where there is a gray zone. A crisis may be perceived by some and not by others depending on the point of view of the observer. As an example, a physician may feel that an individual who is in metabolic alkalosis is in a medical crisis but the given individual may feel they are not.

They may say, "But I feel fine, doctor." Another situation may be that a patient is desperately afraid for their life due to symptoms of palpitations but the doctor, due to EKG tracings confirming a non-life-threatening cause for these symptoms, feels they are not. It is important to know the level of fear or lack of fear in those we care for.

What Is a Medical Crisis?

A crisis, as defined for our purposes, is any situation that is or could become life threatening and lead to sudden death. It could also be any situation that could result in devastating consequences just short of death. Examples of these could be someone experiencing an irreversible drug-induced coma, brain damage, kidney or liver failure, severe cardiac compromise, or suicide attempt to name a few.

A *medical crisis* can be defined as any very serious or critical situation evolving primarily from medical origins. Of course, medical crises may develop from psychological and social origins with self-harm or a violent assault being examples.

What Is Not a Medical Crisis

Situations that might not meet the criteria for medical crisis would be a mildly decreased potassium serum level, runs of a few PVCs with no symptoms of shortness of breath, chest pain, or syncope. We need to be made aware that these seemingly "safe" symptoms and lab values can evolve into a critical, life-threatening situation, literally in a heartbeat. These minor indications of health compromise should be closely paid attention to.

Running on Empty

A car can drive as fast and as effectively on an ounce of gasoline as it can on a full tank. Just by looking at how well a car is driving, however, offers no prediction of how much fuel is left or when it will just stop having run out of gas. When a car completely runs out of gas it stops running immediately. Cars do, however, have a reliable fuel gauge that can show the amount of reserve remaining and give warning well ahead of time of an impending empty fuel tank.

Those with eating disorders often seem to be able to go-go-go right up to the moment their bodies fail. The difference between a car's functioning and a human's is that humans can *compensate* for many declining resources (depleting electrolytes, minerals, hydration) and function (failing cardiac or renal function). This is called homeostasis. Unlike a car, there are no gauges on humans to indicate the degree of declining reserve.

Laboratory and imaging screening do provide somewhat reliable values that can be followed to determine the progression of treatment success or lack of success. While the number values of laboratory investigations are accurate, their ability to indicate a critical event is not. Quoting Hamlet, "Ay, there's the rub."

Clinicians need to be aware that seemingly minor declining laboratory values are not the beginning of the decline of an electrolyte or mineral level but an indication of the body's lack of ability to keep compensating. Essentially they are indicators that the electrolyte or mineral in question is nearing depletion. That is, it is on reserve. Also unpredictable is how much reserve there is or how much further the body will be able to keep compensating. Be aware that seemingly early or minimal body depletions could further decompensate to *lethal values virtually the same day.*

For those who are chronically starved or who chronically use purging methods, the body tends to compensate and adjust to a new homeostasis as nutrients diminish. This only happens to a degree but then there is a limit at which the body can no longer compensate.

The difference between those with eating disorders and those with many other illnesses is that individuals with other health issues tend to feel worse, function worse, and physically look worse. This goes for health problems such as the flu, liver or kidney disease, some cancers, congestive heart failure, and so forth. Those with eating disorders often function at a high level, show up for work or school and can balance many life tasks while being at risk of dying of sudden cardiac death at any moment.

Because of compensating for nutrient deficits, the body slowly becomes depleted of them to a level that at times seems unbelievable that anyone could still remain alive.

The human body follows laws of physics as does any other living creatures, material objects or invisible forces such as gravity, magnetism, or galactic radiation. The human body, however, can seem to defy these laws as we observe in disbelief how anyone can starve to such extremes.

A single laboratory value does not indicate whether a given blood component is stable, increasing or decreasing and what the reserve of it is in organs or has been third spaced. It also does not tell you when the body will no longer compensate and result in death. There need to be frequent serial lab values to get a better picture of any risks.

Expect the Unexpected

When dealing with those with eating disorders expect the unexpected. Regardless of how prepared we feel we are, critical events often happen when we least expect them. All the anticipation and preparedness cannot predict the when, where or even how the crisis will appear. There are too many unknowns or variables that cannot be accounted for in a given unforeseen moment in any particular individual.

Put Drug and Alcohol Abuse at the Top of Compounding Risks

Regardless of overt high-risk eating disorder behaviors with supporting investigative values or even relatively lower risk indicators, illicit drug and alcohol abuse can raise the potential for mortality multifold. It does this by various means.

They can decrease *inhibitions* that would otherwise prevent self-harm behaviors including suicide. Driving while intoxicated, cutting, burning or overdosing are a few self-destructive behaviors. Individuals can certainly die from a direct drug overdose but combining drugs or alcohol with medications such as sedatives, antipsychotics, anti-nauseants, and others can create a compounding depression of the respiratory center of the brain or compromise cardiac function to a lethal end.

Aside from medical and suicide risks, drugs and alcohol can create strife in individual's social functioning, ability to make appropriate judgments, and overall cognitive functioning. What may result is decreasing capacity to concentrate, organize, and complete tasks. This in turn can significantly amplify low self-esteem, hopelessness, helplessness as well as social isolation. Financial destitution may be a risk. Some may be easily taken advantage of by others including exchanging sex for drugs or sexual assault.

The bottom line is, drugs and alcohol can create a mood state and a social environment that help to maintain a grinding destructive course making efforts for recovery and advancement with life goals impossible. Taking drugs or alcohol to cope with an already difficult life is like drilling holes in the hull of a sinking ship with the expectation of letting water out in order to save ones self.

Minor Signs and Symptoms May Be a Harbinger for Catastrophe

We normally worry about the most extremes of lab values, EKG reports as well as medical imaging findings or extremes of physical symptoms. Lesser or seemingly minimal investigation finding or symptoms tend to be allocated to the "not serious" box in our clinical minds. For those with eating disorders, it is prudent to make note of any and all minor medical concerns and keep them *up front and center all of the time.*

The reasons for keeping a sharp eye on *minimal medical indicators* – signs, symptoms, or medical investigations – in those with eating disorders are:

- Minor drops in lab values may be an indication of a major total body decline of electrolytes and minerals after which critical or even lethal drops may develop in very short periods of time.
- Major escalation of eating disorder behaviors may develop unexpectedly that could significantly escalate worsening of medical lab values and symptoms.

- Regardless of the reported lab values for minerals and electrolytes, remaining stores of these cannot be estimated on a person-to-person basis. Each person's reserves may be very different from others and even from time to time in themselves.
- Any individual's capacity to decompensate is unpredictable and can't be assumed. I've seen individuals who have relatively "safe" lower levels of potassium (2.9 mmol/L) develop potentially lethal cardiac rhythms such as torsades de pointe while another with overtly critical values (1.5 mmol/L) is asymptomatic. Lethal risks may not be created in any one individual's lab values but in combination with other compromised values. That is, a combination of low potassium, magnesium, bicarbonate, and elevated sodium may create higher risks than any single low value.
- Some individuals are less likely to follow treatment recommendations such as taking supplements or following-up with caregivers.
- The high functioning ability of many with severe nutrition restriction and extremes of purging and other eating disorder behaviors give clinicians a subconscious false sense of individuals "doing OK."
- Those who abuse drugs and alcohol may be at higher risk overall but as clinicians, we are not likely to be aware of active substance abuse. Polypharmacy will escalate risks as well.
- Undiagnosed preexisting cardiac anomalies may be present that can place individuals at higher risk of sudden cardiac failure.
- A ravished body from nutrition deficits may be more susceptible to overdosing or triggering cardiac excitability even with recommended dosages of prescription or over the counter medications.
- Those with a history of severe starvation plus purging and other eating disorder behaviors are at high risk of *refeeding syndrome.*

Seemingly Predictable Behavior Patterns Cannot Be Trusted to Not Change at Any Moment

The more we work with our patients, the more we likely will feel we understand or truly know an individual's behaviors and can count on them being utilized week after week and month after month. In a number of individuals this may be true but we never really know for sure.

Triggers-Trigger-Triggers

Eating disorder behaviors and attitudes may be triggered without any identifiable cause. Individuals may say "It just happens for no reason." Often, though, there are obvious and predictable reasons. Examples being, binge eating may be triggered by the sight of food; vomiting may be triggered by bingeing and exercise may be triggered by guilt associated with feeling fat.

Laxative use may be triggered by someone standing on a scale and not liking what the scale reads.

Triggers may be caused by *emotions, other eating disorder behaviors,* and *physical symptoms* as well as *life situations.* Critical comments by others, media images or a perceived critical stare by a stranger may be triggering.

Roll-Over Effect

Eating disorders can begin with a single eating disorder behavior triggered by overt body image control desires then evolve from there to become more engrained and long-term. They can also develop out of a set of progenitor attitudes and behaviors that have nothing to do with body image dissatisfaction but then eventually *roll-over* into seedling eating disorder attitudes and behaviors leading to the adoption of a full-on eating disorder. It's as if the raw ingredients of a growing fear of becoming fat, positive feedback for losing weight, a need to feel accomplished at something and envy by others of weight loss then steep or meld together to unwittingly form an eating disorder. The person essentially adopts a kind of Stockholm Syndrome to these destructive influences. Some will say that the eating disorder just came from nowhere – that it was just there one day. Examples of this are as follows.

Individuals who *lose weight* for any reason but do not have significant body image control issues may be at risk of adopting eating disorder attitudes and behaviors. Those that lose weight due to illness, increased physical activity including exercise or "healthy dieting" may receive compliments that they have never had before such as "Do you ever look good" or "How did you lose weight? I can never seem to be able to do that." Where one may have never thought of themselves as overweight or fat, they may develop a mindset that others must have seen them as overweight or fat before weight loss. These accolades will come across as relaying envy and implying the individual has control over weight and food that others have not been able to achieve. A sense of superior will power, when it comes to eating and controlling weight, can be perceived. To keep the accolades coming, one might wish to maintain their low weight status and continue pursuing further weight loss. Although attaining a weight loss goal may be rewarding at first, people usually again feel fat and wish to further lose weight hoping to feel thin at a still lower weight. Weight loss, regardless of how much, tends to not provide individuals a lasting sense of having arrived at a low enough weight. Some may lose 30, 50, a 100 lbs or more and still feel fat. Some will feel fattest at their lowest weight.

Physical illnesses that can lead to weight loss have been listed elsewhere. Mental illnesses such as obsessive compulsive disorder, anxiety, depression, or bipolar disorder may lead to loss of appetite, obsessions regarding food selection such a food aversions, phobias or superstitions – all of these not being connected to body image or weight control initially. Weight loss due to mental illness may lead to fear of becoming fat if nutrition improves, therefore, possibly leading to adopting deliberate weight loss behaviors. Weight loss for any reason may trigger hunger and, thus, uncontrollable drives to eat leading to unexpected weight gain that, in turn, may lead frantically to weight loss behaviors.

Eating Disorders Are Upside Down and Backward From Most Other Medical and Psychological Conditions

There are a number of confounding or confusing factors that seem to fly in the face of good old-fashioned logic.

Individuals Are Typically Very Competent

What gives clinicians as well and family and friends a false sense of security, that the one with an eating disorder is doing "OK," is that they often function well. They seem to function well at many levels. As mentioned above, they can often attend school or work fulltime, attain high academic marks, or perform to a high degree at work. They seem clear thinking and are quick in thought. Organizational skills may be top notch. From a personality perspective, they may be able to work well with a team and may be well liked and deemed competent by coworkers and those in charge. As clinicians we have to be alert to the idea we may be getting acclimatized or "used to" this competence and ignore possible underlying critical medical or mental risks.

What adds to this complacency of clinicians maintaining a sharp focus on potential high risks is that this high functioning can go on for *years* and even *decades*. We adapt to it. The prolonged lack of the individual making efforts to make positive changes toward recovery and the accompanying persistent high functioning drains us of the capacity to stay in a constant state of attention to potential critical risks.

Individuals are Often Very Physically Active Then Just Drop Dead

When reviewing coroner's reports, without exception, all those that died were leading fully active lives. They were either attending college or working on a day-to-day basis, or possibly training in a sport. Death came without any obvious cause in the given moment. One was playing a game of tennis while another was teaching a high-school class when she instantly died. Others were university or high-school students leading seemingly normal, active lives, when one died while watching TV and another died while kissing her boyfriend good night. Some died from suicide without any forewarning.

Physically, the severely medically compromised can perform as well as anyone else with regard to walking, jogging, driving a car or competing successfully in sport. Some will perform with more vim and vigor than those who are considered healthy. We may think "Where do you get all your energy?" Emaciated individuals appear to accomplish physical capabilities far beyond what they should be able to. This is all possible and they still can die in an instant.

Signs and Symptoms Are Often Absent or Minimal Before Death

Likely with those mentioned above, they did not have any significant physical signs or symptoms of note. Recent laboratory investigations may have likely not been carried out or recent values may have been of minimal concern. Individuals may not have followed-up with recommended treatment options regardless of severity of report values.

Individuals May Be Very Aware of Risks But Continue to Pursue a Destructive Course

It is natural for us to assume that those with problems, health or otherwise, will want to make efforts to improve their situation so that they will not suffer the consequences of these difficulties. Humans tend to be survivors and we expect most to want to rise from the ashes as it were. This attitude is especially strong with regard to high functioning and high achieving individuals. It seems illogical or a "waste" that those with great potential would deliberately or inadvertently *sabotage* their own recovery.

There may be many reasons individuals *sabotage* their recovery efforts. Below are just a few.

Fear of Success

For many with eating disorders, there is often a pressure to be successful. It may have been put there by others, by themselves, or both. Because individuals have been seen to be exceptional academically, in sports or the arts or in personal appearance, standards to maintain excellence are encouraged. These pressures may be unwanted and feared. They become afraid to let family, friends, teachers, or coaches down. When someone has an eating disorder they can use it as a reason to not have to maintain a level of competency and even to "let go" of having to be successful. The eating disorder presents the image of illness where others cannot expect them to pursue academics, a career, or other goal-oriented ventures.

Fear of Failure

For some, failure is not an option whether it has to do with meeting eating disorder goals or academic excellence. Failure may be taken very hard largely due to an individual's *self-worth* being tied up with the perceived success of meeting eating disorder expectations including and especially weight goals. Similarly, receiving an A in an exam may bring a great sence of failure and self-loathing when, in fact, an A+ had been hoped for.

Fear of Losing Control

Many with eating disorders would say that the heart of what drives eating disorder pursuits is *control*. Control of what? Some individuals might say they want control in every situation of their life. Another may say she wants *control of just one thing* as she feels she has no control over anything else. Losing control of eating disorder goals is just another form of failure.

Perfectionism, People Pleasing, and Hypersensitivity

This personality triad of is shared by many with eating disorders. These traits can serve as an asset but may get some into trouble.

Perfectionism may create unrealistic expectations of themselves as well as of others. They may procrastinate or not show up for exams or job interviews due to fear of failing.

People pleasing and hypersensitivity may make some vulnerable to being taken advantage of by others or easily emotionally hurt. There may be a constant fear of losing approval by others or hurting their feelings. The eating disorder may provide a sense of maintaining perfection when they cannot achieve this elsewhere. Perfection in controlling food utilization and weight control become ends in themselves or endpoints.

Control Anxiety and Other Emotions

An eating disorder may bring some relief from anxiety and other emotions – a kind of *coping mechanism*. That is, it is a way to control emotions to some degree. The eating disorder may act as a *distraction* from life stressors or provide a relatively *safe place*. The idea of giving up an eating disorder causes great stress or anxiety in many. Without it "How will I cope?"

Fear of Losing Their Identity

Those with eating disorders may find their whole identity is wrapped up in their eating disorder. This identity is not just in their capacity to meet weight goals but in how the rest of the world perceives them. They may become known only for their eating disorder or that's how they may feel. Some with eating disorders may fear that if they give up the eating disorder, others will not know how to perceive them or relate to them. This is akin to a star athlete, who may have been known for being an Olympic contender but then does not make it to the Olympics. The athlete may feel like a failure in the eyes of others and becomes ignored because of their lack of accomplishment. Some failed athletes have to face the insensitive comments by others such as "What went wrong? We were counting on you." During the Vietnam war, soldiers would feel like heroes having served in such a dangerous war and expected a hero's welcome when returning home. Instead, they discovered that they would be called "baby burners" when they returned. Their hoped for identity as a hero had been decimated by a cruel change in the American public's attitude toward the veterans of that time.

Fear of Losing All the Attention They Have Been Receiving Because of the Eating Disorder.

Although the attention that is given to someone with an eating disorder is usually unwanted, it is a kind of attention most likely have never had before. Some may be in denial, or just not want parents or doctors to fuss over their eating disorder behaviors, attitudes, or weight loss. It is attention nonetheless. This sometimes constant and intense attention from others becomes a reward in itself. It can be craved and sought after. A fear of lack of attention could mean that others have given up on them or, possibly, that they are perceived to be recovering, gaining weight, or becoming fat.

Denial

Denial of having an eating disorder, or that it is harmful may be a reason some may not make efforts to recover including improving nutrition. This is similar to an alcoholic who refuses to seek treatment because they feel there isn't a problem in the first place. "Why work on something that does not exist?" Denial may be experienced by those with eating disorders, family, partners as well as caregivers.

Denial may be with regard to the following.

- Denial that an eating disorder exists at all
- Even if the eating disorder is acknowledged, it is not seen as serious
- Denial that treatment options will work
- Denial that the eating disorder is chronic and that it may and will likely take longer than expected for treatment to work
- Caregivers do not believe in treatment course
- A caregiver denies a given individual has a chance of recovery

Denial may be in regard to the one with the eating disorder, family members or individuals within a treatment team. On the other hand, some may be on board in recognition of the eating disorder and treatment course.

Fear of Being Normal

An eating disorder sets individuals apart from family, friends, and peers. They become "exceptional" or special in their own eyes and possibly in the eyes of others. Because the eating disorder gives them a new *status* or *identity*, they may fear being normal without it. Being normal may be deemed the same as being mediocre or unimportant.

Desire to Not Be Deemed a Sexual Being

Sexuality may be feared by some with eating disorders. This may be because the individual does not want to face adult responsibilities which includes being sexual. All too many with eating disorders have a history of sexual assault. As a result of this, being perceived as a sexual being becomes a repugnant option. Severe weight loss or major weight gain can send signals to others that his person does not wish to be sexual or is undesirable as a sexual respondee. Extreme body shapes such as being cachectic or overweight can make individuals feel they are unattractive or *unsexy* to others which may be their intended goal. Some may choose to appear androgynous. Those with an emaciated body may experience significant hormonal shifts which inhibit sexual feelings.

Fear of Becoming Fat

Certainly, especially early on in recovery efforts, recovering means gaining weight and becoming fat. Weight gain or the lack of ability to lose weight is the apex of feared outcomes with recovery. Major resistance to improved nutrition and the resulting weight increase is at the forefront of not wanting to recover.

Desire to Be Punished

To some, the eating disorder is a form of punishment. A sense of "I don't deserver better." prevails. *Shame* and *guilt* may be at the heart of wanting and needing to be punished.

Guilt and Shame

Guilt and shame are powerful driving forces for many with eating disorders. These emotions further help to erode an esteem that is already fragile.

The following are only a few possibilities for which one would feel guilt or shame.

- Disappointing parents in regard to not being accomplished enough in areas such as academics, sports, the arts, or career as examples
- Not being as, and especially, more accomplished than peers in regard to popularity, thinness, academics, sports or the arts
- Not being a good person. Guilt or shame may arise from not taking more responsibility for global warming, animal cruelty or visiting their grandmother more in the retirement home. Some will have guilt seemingly on all fronts
- Not looking attractive enough
- Being overweight
- Not being thin enough
- Getting a "bad mark" in an exam or university course. A bad mark may be an A- to some

Fear of Losing a Life-Line

The eating disorder to some is more than a weight and body image control device or coping mechanism for all sorts of concerns. To some, it is a life-line. That is, it is the most important or only thing that keeps them alive. The threat of taking the eating disorder away can remove the only device that is keeping them alive.

When working with someone we are trying to help recover, make sure that they do not perceive it as taking way their only life-line. Some will become suicidal while others will suicide. I have asked patients to actually keep their eating disorder behavior active in the mean time to prevent suicide. That is, to give permission, as it were, to engage in their eating disorder attitudes and behaviours at least until acute suicide ideation passes. There is no harm in putting recovery plans on hold in order to save someone's life. Close medical and psychological monitoring are a must.

Lack of Will, Mental and Physical Energy to Maintain Efforts

Maintaining an eating disorder as well as efforts toward recovery takes seemingly unrelenting effort day after day, month after month and sometimes year after year. It is like a marathon that never ends. Chronic mental and physical exhaustion invariably sets in. Asking someone to make more effort toward recovery is like asking a marathon runner to acquire the physical and head energy to continue after a 26 mile run with no end in site. Periods of "time out" or coasting time are essential to recovery for some. Athletic coaches build in rest periods or recovery time for competitive athletes after a day of hard physical input. Recovery efforts must be paced.

Lack of Success With Recovery Efforts

Working toward recovery after a long time of maintaining an eating disorder is frustrating and exhausting at best. Having done all this work and then finding that recovery efforts are not working can destroy hope. Clients and families need to be informed that a seeming lack of recovery now may be looked at as a plateau that needs to be ridden out. It is to be looked at as a necessary part of recovery and may be treated as *time out*.

Anxiety, Depression, or Psychosis

These mental health issues fan the flames of destructive drives. Worsening anxiety, depression, or psychosis may diminish the will to have to deal with them. Recover hopes become a mirage.

Being Too "Drugged-up"

Those who take sedating medications whether prescribed, over the counter or in the form of street drugs may find it difficult if not impossible to attend to recovery efforts. The capacity to *concentrate* or *focus* on the multitude of confounding factors needed to infuse recovery efforts may be unrealistic with a drugged mind.

Fear of Growing Up and Becoming a Responsible Adult

A real fear for some people is that of having to "grow up" or taking on adult responsibilities as noted above in *Desire to Not Be Deemed a Sexual Being*.

Adulthood involves having to take on responsibilities not expected of children and young teenagers. These responsibilities are to make their own decisions, finish an education, obtain a job and be competent at it, socialize with adults, engage in relationships as well as take on debt and so forth. Some prefer to remain in the body of a child and not have adult responsibilities.

Superstition or Fear Something Horrible Will

Some fear something terrible will happen to others if they do not keep up eating disorder or possibly other rituals. It's a kind of superstition. They may be afraid for themselves for the same reasons. Forgetting or deliberately not engaging in eating disorder behaviors is akin to stepping on a sidewalk crack that will "break your mother's back." Some rituals may be linked to obsessive-compulsive behaviors. Rituals may meet eating disorder, superstitious and obsessive-compulsive disorder needs all at the same time or at varying times depending on the trigger.

Continuing Abusive Relationships and Other Harsh Life Stressors

Ongoing abusive relationships whether with a partner, roommates, co-workers, or family can hinder recovery efforts. Individuals need to be removed from these toxic relationships for their own mental health and safety as well as to help pave the way for steady recovery efforts. Cyberbullying is a very real source of abuse.

History of Sexual, Physical, or Emotional Abuse

Experiences of sexual, physical, or emotional abuse all tie in to a poor self-esteem. They may be at the heart of what drives the eating disorder in the first place. Regardless, people must be removed from ongoing threats of these abuses and, to some degree, address their importance in how these experiences have shaped their lives including the possible influence on the eating disorder, moods, relationships as well as drug or alcohol use. All abuses may drive suicidal thoughts and actions.

Drug and Alcohol Abuse

Drug and alcohol abuse may put individuals at the *highest suicide risk* regardless of how severe their eating disorder behaviors and medical risks are.

Dementia

Early dementia creates all kinds of confusion prior to a proper diagnosis. For some with a developing eating disorder and evolving dementia, major body image discontent can seemingly appear from nowhere. Concern over food and food restriction may ensue. The connection between dementia and the subsequent development of an eating disorder is a mystery. Prior to dementia, could the individual have had feelings of being overweight but had never expressed this to family and friends or acted on these feelings by dieting or engaging other weight losing behaviors? Or, does body image dissatisfaction evolve from the dementia state? Does dementia remove normal inhibitions including those that affect undesirable concerns about weight? This is for geriatric researchers to determine.

Peaceful Coexistence With Eating Disorder

A significant motivation for maintaining effective eating disorder attitudes and behaviors is for one to adopt a *peaceful coexistence* with their eating disorder. That is, the eating disorder behaviors are working enough to sustain adequate weight and body image control yet not creating medical or psychological signs that can be noticed by others. Medical signs would be stumbling, falling, fainting, or increasing weight loss that family or professional caregivers would notice. They glide through their life harboring an active eating disorder without others being alerted to worrisome health concerns. Individuals find a happy balance between effective eating disorder efforts and giving the impression of being healthy enough to not be noticed. This helps to keep others from feeling they have to interfere and hopefully leave the individual alone. Not all, but many do fear for their lives as they know how dangerous developing a medical compromise can be. They reach a point of compromise where they are looking into a catastrophic abyss but not falling into it. A dubious balancing act at best.

A major result of this peaceful coexistence is that people get lost to follow-up and can drift from medical, psychological, and family support quite unnoticed. Because of the perception they are "doing OK," it's easy for caregivers and loved ones to feel they can loosen up with having to pay as close attention. The "worry guard" goes down. It is, however, just as important to have close follow-up when individuals are actually doing better or seemingly doing better.

Contributions to Risk

Addressing these factors may be the best way to decrease risk.

A Theory of Accumulative Risks

Although not supported by research yet, it is likely that risks accumulate with the *intensity* to which a given eating disorder behavior is used, the *number of different eating disorder behaviors* engaged as well as the addition of evolving *medical risks*. These medical risks may already be known or, indeed, occult. *Suicidal risk* potentially compounds even further the accumulated risk.

Why it is important to be aware of possible accumulated risks is that any one risk may not seem very threatening by itself. However, when compounded with a number of other risks, may in total become serious.

Intent

Regardless of what individuals say to you about their eating disorder goals, such as weight loss, their *true intent* or degree of dogged determination to achieve this goal is what is most important. One may say she wants to lose 30 lbs, but has never been able to lose more than 15 lbs. Another, however, may say she wants to lose 30 lbs and has a history of losing 50 lbs. This last person has a proven track record of major weight loss and has a tried and true experience as to how to accomplish this. Both individuals have the same weight loss goal but one likely has a greater achievable intent.

Intent may be able to be guessed at not just by previous successes at weight loss but by the choices of eating disorder behaviors and extremes of their use. One individual may want to lose 30 lbs by restricting daily food intake to 1200 calories and exercising by walking two hours a day. Another may set a daily nutrition intake of 500 calories, vomit 20 times daily and will not stop vomiting until she sees blood in her vomitus. She also takes 30 Ex-Lax tables daily and goes to the gym for a hard five hour workout every day. The same weight loss goal – different intent.

Even if weight loss is minimal with ones best efforts, the extremes of eating disorder behaviors and medical risks are far more important to pay attention to. The degree of intended weight loss has importance for sure and can become critical. However, the methods of achieving weight loss and level of medical compromise require close monitoring. Some with eating disorders may be in a normal weight range but use extremes of behaviors and may have critical life-threatening metabolic and cardiac compromise.

One thing to consider regarding intent is that in spite of our best efforts in assessing this, we really do not have many reliable parameters with which to do so. There are those with seemingly milder eating disorder behaviors that have been able to achieve inordinate weight loss and lethal medical compromise. Regardless of our assessment of someone's intents to lose weight, assume a worst-case scenario is possible right from first contact.

Eating Disorder Behavior Specific Risks

Multiple Eating Disorder Behaviors

The more kinds of eating disorder behaviors one utilizes may, in theory, raise risks for medical as well as emotional and financial, relationship and other compromises. While some may utilize one eating disorder behavior at a given time, others may utilize dozens concurrently. Some eating disorder behaviors may be added to an already established set of behaviors. I knew a patient with thirty active eating disorder behaviors as well as ten others she would rely on from time to time.

The more different kinds of eating disorder behaviors one uses, there will be an additive risk from each. As an example, if someone vomits twice daily there will be X amount of risk including and especially medical ones. If the use of laxatives is then added to the regime, medical risk may be elevated. Adding to this diuretic use and fluid overloading, again, medical risk can be expected to be escalated further. Vomiting, laxative, and diuretic use as well as fluid overloading each has a risk of its own for creating metabolic dysfunction. Cumulatively, risk may escalate. Adding cocaine, opioid, and alcohol use plus accelerated weight loss may aggravate an existing mitral value prolapse and ramp up the risk of lethal cardiac dysrhythmias. That is, the risk of sudden cardiac death.

Aside from medical risks, the risks for depression, anxiety, psychosis, social isolation, relationship strife, unemployment as well as a myriad of other social ills are possible.

Increased Use of Each Eating Disorder Behavior

While the accumulated utilization of multiple eating disorder behaviors may increase risk, so may the escalated use of each behavior. There are various methods of increasing utilization.

INCREASING FREQUENCY

Many behaviors may be increased with the frequency of their use. Someone who takes laxatives once a week may increase their use to daily. Someone who vomits once a day may increase this to four times a day. Increasing the frequency of use of behaviors increases the number of times used in a given time period but may not increase the total number used for any session of use. As an example, one may typically vomit 16 times in day over a 12-hour period. Increasing the frequency of vomiting episodes to 16 times in four hours then vomiting no more, increases the frequency but not total daily count.

INCREASING VOLUME

Volume increases may be possible with binge eating where, as an example, an individual binges on a pint of ice cream in one sitting then increases this to two quarts a sitting. Some who fluid load on a single glass of water may increase this to several glasses at a time.

INCREASING NUMBER

Examples of increasing numbers used are:

- Increasing vomiting from once a week to 10 times a day
- Increasing using 2 laxative tablets a day to 30
- Increasing pushups from 10 daily to 100 daily

INCREASING LENGTH OF TIME

Some eating disorder behaviors used may be increased by the length of time they are utilized. Increasing time length for use of an eating disorder may increase the number, frequency, and sometimes volume of use.

INCREASING INTENSITY

Some will increase the intensity of use of a given eating disorder. Examples of this are:

- Running faster or doing sit-ups faster
- Vomiting more forcefully by using emetics instead of fingers
- Lifting heavier weights
- Running or swimming farther

While most eating disorder behaviors that increase in frequency, number, volume or length of time could increase medical risks, restricting or lessening eating adds to risk as well.

Extreme Use of Each Eating Disorder Behavior

Though increased use of eating disorder behaviors could increase risk, the *extreme* use of these behaviors ramp up potential risk multifold.

While increasing vomiting from twice daily to five times daily or increasing daily laxative use from 5 tablets daily to 20 may be riskier, some vomit 50, 60 or 80 times a day or take 300 Ex-Lax tablets a day. These extreme behaviors do occur and clinicians must be aware of this in given individuals.

Escalating Endpoints

Increasing the use of any eating disorder behavior is likely done for the purpose of *speeding up* the rate of achieving whatever any eating disorder goal may be.

Increasing the use of an eating disorder *plus escalating endpoints* further compounds risk. These endpoints, as mentioned elsewhere, can lead to see blood or experience palpitations while vomiting, lose more weight or to become thinner.

Kinds of Eating Disorder Behaviors and Relative Risk

Not all eating disorder behaviors carry the same risk. Having said this, because there has not been any research into *relative risk* for any given eating disorder behavior we cannot make accurate assumptions regarding risk.

As an example, vomiting using a cardiotoxic emetic will likely provide more medical risk than chewing gum used to suppress appetite. An unknown here is how much a seemingly minor behavior such as chewing gum may add just that little extra push into medical compromise given other behaviors have created the major risks. If chewing gum can aid in someone losing 30 lbs due to restricting food intake, then this significant weight loss alone can create medical risk by itself. A significant weight loss on top of a threatening metabolic abnormality with associated risk of a lethal dysrhythmia could realistically cause sudden cardiac death. One behavior may act as an *igniter* to others.

Combinations of Eating Disorder Behaviors to Create the Same Effect

Some eating disorder behaviors have the *same intended effect* as others. As examples, chewing gum, smoking, sucking on sugarless candies, appetite suppressants, watching TV and walking the dog all have the intended use of suppressing appetite or distracting from eating. They all are intended to restrict food intake. Exercising, taking metabolism boosters, smoking cigarettes, cocaine use, or sweating in a sauna are all utilized to increase metabolism in order to burn calories.

Duration of Eating Disorder

Is having an eating disorder for a long period of time a predictor for chronicity or lethality?

One definition of *chronic diseases* can be defined broadly as conditions that last one year or more and require ongoing medical attention or limit activities of daily living or both. Another definition defines a health condition as chronic if it lasts three months or longer. I would add to this that even if activities of daily living are not affected, symptoms may persist for a prolonged period of time. An example of this would be chronic back pain where by the individual can fully function regardless of ongoing pain. This condition may present constantly or on and off. Eating disorders, by nature, are typically chronic. Though eating disorder behaviors and attitudes tend to be ongoing, they may be reoccurring or intermittent. Because an individual with an eating disorder does not receive medical attention or daily activities do not appear affected, this does not mean they do not have a serious and chronic illness.

Family History of Eating Disorders

Genetic research has shown that there is a strong genetic component to developing eating disorder traits in some families. In other words, there may be a congenital predisposition to individuals developing an eating disorder from conception. I have seen a family where the mother had had an eating disorder – bulimia – when she was younger. All three of her daughters acquired bulimia in their teens as well. In this situation there had not been any eating disorder triggers such as expressed personal body size concerns or comments about others body sizes or shapes passed on from the mother when the girls grew up. She was also very careful to not comment on food choices nor discussed eating disorders in the home.

Ever-Changing Risk Factors

It's hard enough to follow any single risk factor let alone multiple risk factors at the same time. Complicating things further is that various *risk factors come and go* while *new ones may emerge* seemingly from nowhere. This is similar to the Whac-A- Mole game where mechanized moles pop up and as you knock one down, another emerges from somewhere else.

Risk factors created by eating disorder behaviors or from other sources come and go with changing eating disorder behaviors and other risk provoking situations. Adding to already existing risks may be *new* risk factors that *compound risks* and further confuse clinicians. Be aware of the chance for changing or morphing risk factors.

Toxic Eating Disorder Peer Relationships

Sometimes those with eating disorders rely on each other to motivate themselves to push the envelop for weight loss and body image control. They form a kind of peer support group but not for recovery sake. Competition for weight loss or extremes of eating disorder behavior use may emerge. Each seeks bragging rights to outdo the other. In other words, they encourage others to be sick. These toxic relationships are notoriously common in eating disorder treatment facilities. They also exist in the community sometimes as a result of patients having met while forming a friendship in a treatment facility then carrying their motivational relationship out of hospital or residential care facility. Separating individuals in treatment centers so they do not form toxic relationships may be required.

Unfortunately, because of social networking individuals from around the world can meet on a blog site, Facebook, Instagram, Twitter and other networking formats. These networking sites have been referred to as *Pro-Ana* and *Pro-Mia* sites.

Pro-Ana and Pro-Mia Networking Sites

Pro-ana and pro-mia internet sites are typically created by those with eating disorders. They encourage others with eating disorders to pursue often extremes of eating disorder behaviors and weight loss goals. These sites are toxic and may encourage self-harm behaviors including suicide. These sites may be shut down legally as any internet link that can hurt minors is illegal. The problem is, those that get removed from one site on the internet will likely reemerge somewhere else.

Disfiguration

Those with eating disorders already have a hypersensitivity to how they look with regard to body size and shape. Disfiguration of any part of the body even if hidden by clothing just creates more grief.

Examples of disfiguring conditions are individuals with neurofibroma tumors or the surgical scars from having these tumors removed. Bad plastic surgery outcomes of the face, breast augmentation or reduction, liposuction or tummy tucks are a few. Botched labiaplasty surgery can cause grievous regret.

Anyone planning any cosmetic surgery should be informed of the possibility of poor outcomes and if they think that they could not live with the final results should seriously consider postponing surgery or forgetting about surgical options all together. Individuals may have to deal with bad surgical outcomes that may not be reversible or even improved upon satisfactorily. Disfiguration may be permanent. The cost of reversing poor surgical outcomes may be prohibitive.

Ongoing and Compounding Stressors

As medical conditions compound recovery efforts for those with eating disorders, so do additional life stresses. Stressors may come from employment, school, debt, difficult relationships, ongoing failures, bullying and so on. Non-eating disorder life stressors can each become the focus of ones life, taking away attention to eating disorder recovery. Not knowing where next month's rent money is coming from, how one is going to insure their car or be able to pay for food will be one's primary focus in life if unemployed. Being caught up in an abusive relationship will require consuming attention. When building a treatment plan for an individual's eating disorder recovery, be aware of all other important life stressors so as to include viable solutions to their resolve. Other professional resources may be required such as drug and alcohol counselors, family therapists, sexual assault counselors, social workers who can assist with housing and employment concerns, or police to protect against the threat of partner violence.

Not Believing In Recovery

For years I believed that anyone who was coming to see me for their eating disorder must believe in recovery otherwise they would not be coming. Wrong. Individuals may be seeing caregivers and yet not believe they can be helped. Early on in contact with someone, the clinician should enquire as to whether the individual believes they can recover or at least improve. We as professionals should state that we believe in improvement including recovery to help establish an environment of healing.

I have said to individuals that they do not have to necessarily believe in recovery before committing to treatment. Someone does not have to believe that an antibiotic will cure an ear infection. Cure will occur regardless. To some degree, this may be true for recovery from an eating disorder. Evolving trust in caregivers and evidence of even minor successes will help bring faith in the recovery process.

Lack of Hope and Feelings of Hopelessness

Expecting someone to be motivated to recover when they have feelings of hopelessness and helplessness is pretty much pointless. It becomes a "Can lead a horse to water ... ." scenario. A sense of a lack of hope or hopelessness may pervade everything in one's life or may be only in specific areas. Hope needs to be vitalized before there are likely to be gains in treatment. Having said this, moving forward with treatment is essential trusting hope will follow.

Responsibility of Care for Others

Some have to care for others regardless that they themselves may require much care. This is so, of course, when individuals have children to care for. Sometimes someone needs to care for a parent who is ill with a mental or physical condition or who may be a severe alcoholic who cannot take care of themselves. It is not uncommon to hear that those with eating disorders are the "parent of the parents." Parents or others may depend heavily on some to take care of them. It may be necessary to interject support from friends, family or professional caregivers in order to help remove the dependency on those with eating disorders.

Dependence on Eating Disorder to Cope With Life

One of the greatest powers the eating disorder has over any individual is its importance in how they use the eating disorder to cope with life. Some might say the eating disorder is a *crutch* used in many of life situations. Some depend on the eating disorder to be able to function in virtually any situation.

The following are various items for which an eating disorder may be used in order to cope.

A friend

Some will describe their eating disorder as a friend. It is *reliable, familiar* and, in an odd way, they can *trust it.*

Cope with Emotions

The eating disorder becomes a coping mechanism for many undesirable emotions – fear, anger, anxiety, depression, and so on. The focus on meeting eating disorder goals can displace negative emotions at least for a while.

A Distraction From Life Tasks

Life has many expectations. These include having to succeed academically, in a career, dealing with family, a partner and other relationships as well as making a living. The eating disorder can act as a distraction from life tasks.

"It's What I'm Good At."

Some feel the eating disorder is the only thing that they are good at regardless of how accomplished they may be at other things such as academics, athletics, or kindling relationships. Being aware of the eating disorder as a mechanism to cope with many situations will help the clinician to navigate their approach to someone with an eating disorder.

"Must Knows" For Reducing Risks

There are a few items clinicians must know about in order to help anticipate and reduce critical medical risks.

- Expect the unexpected.
- Imagine or try to anticipate the critical medical-worse-case scenarios.
- Develop as complete an understanding as possible of eating disorder behaviors as well as the permutations and combinations of their use.
- Know what triggers eating disorder attitudes and behaviors, emotions as well as physical symptoms. Understand the domino-effect or billiard ball like expression of one trigger upon others. Triggers-trigger-triggers.
- Have a complete, closed loop, follow-up plan anticipating possible gaps in service.
- Engage the services of other clinicians or networks that aid in completing the *treatment loop*.
- Talk to caregivers, family, and other significant others when possible.

Medical Considerations

Drug Reactions and Drug Interactions

Serious drug reactions can result in someone being gun shy with regard to trying new medications. This can be detrimental when an individual requires medication to deal with serious health conditions such as depression, psychosis, gut dysmotility syndrome to name a few. Allergic reactions, serotonin syndrome, tardive dyskinesia, and psychotic reactions are examples of drug reactions. The medication, cisipride, a gastroprokinetic agent, caused lethal dysrhythmias in some with anorexia nervosa and has been taken off the market.

Some drug interactions to be aware of are monoamine oxidase inhibitors in combination with selective serotonin reuptake inhibitors or tricyclic antidepressants. Red wine and cheeses are to be avoided as well. The use of some anticoagulants and acetylsalacylic acid needs to be assessed by knowledgeable clinicians.

Sedating drugs, when added together, can create a multifold sedating effect that is far greater than the individual sedating effect of each by themselves. That is, therapeutic levels of sedating drugs when combined with another can cause unconsciousness or respiratory arrest. Alcohol or narcotics added to prescription or over the counter sedating medications is an example.

Kinds and Degree of Symptoms or Signs

As mentioned elsewhere, individuals may have life-threatening and even lethal health risks without signs or symptoms. Relying on symptoms and signs and the severity with which they may present in order to assess risk is not going to be helpful and can be dangerous. Having said this, if signs and symptoms have been investigated and serious medical risk has been ruled out, pay attention to their increasing frequency and intensity regardless as escalation may be an indication of impending risk.

Coexisting Medical Conditions – Not Caused By Eating Disorder

As if having an eating disorder with the potential medical risks it possesses is not enough, non-eating disorder medical conditions complicates risk and management further.

Any important non-eating disorder related medical condition may command a diligent focus with regard to its management and, therefore, could take away from the attention the eating disorder requires. It also may add a compounding set of risks. This other medical condition may be another burden to cope with. The individual may find having to deal with more than one major health issue is more than they are capable of dealing with. Chronic pain, insulin dependent diabetes mellitis, and inflammatory bowel disease are only a few to mention.

Many coexisting medical conditions may increase risks already created by the eating disorder.

Significant Weight Loss Regardless of Cause

Significant weight loss by itself is a risk factor regardless of cause. Restricting, exercising, purging methods as well as metabolism stimulants all contribute to weight loss. Non-eating disorder causes of weight loss must be considered such as diabetes, hyperthyroidism, malignancies, and other wasting illness.

Defining *significant weight loss* is a challenge. Any weight loss that creates medical compromise has to be considered significant. What may be considered modest weight loss due to other illness could add to the medical risks caused by the eating disorder behaviors themselves. That is, we may not think of 15 lbs weight loss from a normal weight as likely a serious threat by itself but dysrhythmias or syncope may be triggered by this modest drop in weight in some situations. This is akin to "the straw that broke the camel's back." Certainly a 15 lbs loss due to a non-eating disorder illness on top of an already 40 lbs loss due to eating disorder behaviors escalates risk. Weight loss from any cause may amplify the medical risks created by any and all eating disorder behaviors.

Not Taking Medications

Those with eating disorders may be taking medications for any number of reasons. Some of them may be to assist in eating disorder treatment or for other reasons not related to the eating disorder. Depending on the medication and the health issue it is being used for, the degree of consequence for not taking the medication will vary. Consequences may be not at all, minimal or possibly life-threatening. Frequent medication review is essential.

Included in a medication review should be prescribed, over the counter and street drugs used. The use of supplements such as vitamins and minerals as well as herbal and ethnic remedies are to be mentioned. Special diet restrictions should accompany a medication and supplement review. Gluten and dairy free diets may be connected to heath concerns that dictate supplement usage.

Though refusing to take some medications may not cause any serious outcomes, not taking anticoagulants, insulin, anti-seizure medications, antipsychotic, or antidepressant medications as well as several others may be dangerous or even lethal. Declining to use contraceptive methods may lead to unwanted pregnancies.

Refusal to take a medication may be due to the fear of weight gain. Contraceptive methods, antidepressants, and antiseizure and antipsychotic medications are a few.

Medical Conditions That Imitate Eating Disorders

Although it may be obvious to someone with an eating disorder as well as to others that a given individual has an eating disorder, there can be gray zones or outright confusion as to whether someone, indeed, has an eating disorder or not. Some of this confusion comes as many signs and symptoms of other illnesses are identical to those of eating disorders. Confusion comes also with other illnesses coexisting along side an eating disorder. Attributing particular signs or symptoms to an incorrect health issue, either an eating disorder or another illness by mistake, can be dangerous. Following are medical and psychological conditions that can imitate eating disorders.

Any *medical condition* that produces the following symptoms could be confused with someone having an eating disorder.

- Loss of appetite
- Nausea
- Vomiting
- Weight loss
- Chronic abdominal and pelvic pain
- Syncope, stumbling, loss of consciousness
- Any combination of the above

Any *psychological condition* that produces the following symptoms could be confused with someone having an eating disorder.

- Loss of appetite
- Nausea
- Vomiting
- Weight loss
- Food phobias
- Food obsessions
- Obsessive-compulsive disorder
- Selective eating
- Any psychological condition that affects eating or weight control not associated with body image dissatisfaction

These are a few diagnoses that may incorporate one or many of the symptoms above.

- Addison's disease
- Hyperthyroidism
- Insulin-dependent diabetes mellitis
- Malignancies
- Gastrointestinal Disorders

  - Irritable bowel syndrome
  - Inflammatory bowel disease
  - Celiac disease
  - Cholecystitis
  - Malabsorption syndrome
  - Gastrointestinal infections
  - Any condition that causes chronic abdominal and pelvic pain

- Gynecological Disorders

  - Endometriosis
  - Pelvic adhesions
  - Sensitivity to the combined oral contraceptive pill
  - Sensitivity to one's own endogenous estrogen
  - Undiagnosed pregnancy

- Brain tumor
- Dementia

Some of these disorders are mentioned in depth elsewhere.

Mental Health

Mental health issues affect *all* those with eating disorders. After all, eating disorders are classified as mental illnesses. Compounding eating disorder specific mental health issues are often depression and anxiety as well as possibly obsessive-compulsive disorder, bipolar spectrum disorder, and personality disorders. Any mental health diagnoses may accompany an eating disorder. Oppressive mental health concerns need to be addressed concurrently with medical management and eating disorder recovery efforts. Suicide is the number one enemy of many with eating disorders.

Some mental illnesses predate the eating disorder and may thrive regardless of possible eating disorder influences. That is, they can have a life of their own. Preexisting mental illness may, however, be amplified or aggravated by the eating disorder. Of course, eating disorder attitudes and behaviors may also be worsened by mental health stressors. Mental illnesses may present after an eating disorder manifests itself and may go hand in hand with eating disorder dynamics. In this case, mental health may improve as the eating disorder comes to some resolve.

Some May Not Present With Evidence of Predictive Suicidal Risks

Many do not show signs of depression or indicate suicidal tendencies. *Impulsivity* for suicide, other self-harm or dangerous eating disorder behaviors are the scariest part of managing care. The person themselves may not have an awareness of impending impulsive acts.

Accidental Overdose

Never underestimate the chance of an accidental overdose. This will more likely be the result of an *impulsive* and *accidental* overdose. "I just wanted to have a good sleep." may be the response in the ICU the day after such an event. For these individuals, find out if there were any triggers just prior such as bullying, a fight with a parent or a bout of depression and so forth. The trigger may be simply boredom or just a narrow window of opportunity to carry out the overdose when no one is around to observe them. In such a situation, parents may have been briefly out of the home or hospital ward staff were attending to others. Street drugs and alcohol certainly can decrease an individual's inhibitions and judgment.

Self-Harm

Self-harm comes in many forms. Some are not particularly dangerous while others are lethal. We need to be aware of self-harm thoughts and viable behaviors.

Some serious self-harm actions are as follows.

- Drug or alcohol overdose – deliberate or accidental
- Cutting of wrists, carotid artery or femoral artery
- Driving while drunk or stoned
- Hanging
- Drowning
- Hitting ones self
- Phlebotomy
- Caustic enemas
- Several others

Needless to say, many of the above actions may lead to death.

Clinician, Staff, and Treatment Considerations

With the potential for several clinicians and other staff being involved with the care of those with eating disorders, it is little wonder that system glitches occur. When I admitted individuals to a ward for treatment of their eating disorder, I would tell them that there *will be* system upsets so they would be somewhat prepared ahead of time. It was my job to help them navigate the ups and downs of treatment and to stay the course. It is our job to help navigate treatment and act as advocates.

Causes of Incorrect Diagnoses and Inadequate Treatment

There are many sources of communication breakdown or disconnect. Be aware of them.

Splitting

Splitting is a term that is often misunderstood and misused in psychology. In short, it can refer to an individual developing black or white thinking or all or none thinking, splitting of the ego, or a manipulative splitting of staff through false claims. Regardless, its misuse in regard to the care of those with eating disorders can be damaging to patient and caregiver relationships.

Splitting is a common word used in the care of those with eating disorders and is often meant in a derogatory manner. It implies that a patient is deliberately manipulating caregivers by making false claims. As an example, a patient who claims she was to be allowed out on a weekend pass when an order by the attending physician had not been written supporting this claim, may be seen as splitting or manipulating staff for her own end. An individual who balks against receiving 2% milk for breakfast instead of her claim of agreeing with the dietitian to receive 1% milk may be seen as manipulative and unjustly argumentative, and is splitting behavior.

When I was told/informed a patient was splitting by nurses, doctors, or dietitians, I would immediately cross check the patient's claims with staff and 100% of the time, the patient was correct. In the situations mentioned above, the individual was told she was to have a weekend pass but the physician had forgotten to write it in the chart – not that uncommon an error we have all made. With regard to the milk incident, the patient was correct and the dietitian had indeed said 1% was OK for breakfast. Here the dietitian had not conveyed to staff this decision or possibly the staff had not looked for this information that had been clearly stated in the chart.

Regardless of claims by patients and staff to the contrary, confirm with all parties involved the accuracy of their stories and communicate to all concerned a definitive conclusion. This will help reduce tensions between those we are treating and caregivers. Yes, patients can scheme and sometimes do but firm up for sure that they are or are not doing so. Because others have been manipulative does not mean your current client is or will be. If they are, indeed, trying to be manipulative, be kind and understand that these behaviors are a sometimes expected outcome during treatment. Allow and encourage, to some degree, an individual's right in keeping information to themselves or telling white lies. Give pats on the back for coming clean at a later date. This conveys a "go with the flow" attitude. Role-play and put the client in the caregiver role: "What would you think or do in this situation?" Gaining trust is the best way to have clients come clean. We don't berate a patient admitted to the coronary ICU (CICU) for having a string of premature ventricular contractions or angina when we hope they will not occur. Caregivers in CICU would never say "By having angina you are not cooperating with treatment!"

False Assumptions

False assumptions by clinicians can and will lead to misdiagnoses and inappropriate treatment options. Unfortunately there are more incorrect assumptions than hard accurate knowledge, it seems, with regard to eating disorders. We need to be very aware of our own assumptions and make concerted efforts to glean out the bad ones.

False assumptions can be made regarding a whole spectrum of aspects related to individuals with eating disorders. These are made with regard to the misunderstanding of eating disorders generally including eating disorder attitudes and behaviors, motivations, attitudes toward school, work, or careers, relationships as well as emotions, destructive behaviors, and many other related items.

Inappropriate assumptions can be made that someone indeed has an eating disorder based on their behaviors, physical signs, and symptoms that appear eating disorder in nature. This is akin to police assuming someone is intoxicated due to observing an awkward gait and stumbling who, instead, has multiple sclerosis or cerebral palsy. These assumptions are too easy to make including by experts.

Poor Understanding of Eating Disorders

Treatment regimes for eating disorders have been around for over 60 years. The concern is that there has been very poor understanding of eating disorders the whole time. All treatment models have been developed utilizing a very poor knowledge base. While major efforts have been dedicated to various treatments that come and go, attempts to understand eating disorder behaviors, attitudes, and the intricate relationships of these to emotions, social situations, and other dynamics has never evolved to any depth. The only way to learn about eating disorders is to have the skill set to take very precise and detailed eating disorder focused histories. Much of what has to be learned is acquired through experience and a dogged commitment to detail.

Influence From Colleagues and Staff

Those clinicians that we work with by sharing the care of our clients can be of major assistance to our own efforts. However, we have to carefully filter what information we share with them. There are a few reasons for this.

- Because few colleagues have any significant experience with those with eating disorders, their interpretation of what they think they know may be inaccurate.
- Clinical staff may harbor negative biases and inaccurate stereotypic impressions of our clients.
- They may not have the skills to make an accurate diagnosis of an eating disorder or to rule it out.
- Consult notes and discharge summaries may relay incorrect conclusions and may be out of date.

I have witnessed individuals who have been treated year after year for an eating disorder who never had an eating disorder in the first place. This is largely because subsequent treatments by physicians relied on previously available consult notes stating an incorrect diagnosis in the beginning. We tend to rely on the wisdom and accuracy of experts especially in the field of eating disorders. So we tend to assume they are reliable sources and can trust their judgment. Too many errors have been made by experts.

Review all of the information available from colleagues that we have access to but we need to take our own thorough verbal eating disorder assessment as well as obtain a thorough medical assessment through history, physical examination, and review of medical investigations. Collateral information from nurses, dietitians, social workers, and other professionals may be invaluable but screen for accuracy.

Lack of Team Communication

Treatment teams, whether a part of hospital- or community-based programs including residential ones, form the core of professional support. Communication is the key to a cohesive working unit. Communication styles only determine whether the teams work well together or not.

Where communication breaks down is:

- Team members are not on the same page as to how to deliver treatment options
- Treatment options have not been fully decided upon
- Staff shift changes
- Staff don't like working with those with eating disorders
- Staff are dealing with their own issues regarding diet and weight control
- There is not adequate funding for programs
- Physician, dietitian, or other clinician orders are not clearly stated in the charts
- Chart notes have not been entered
- The team does not communicate adequately with the patient or family.
- All of the above!

Although teams are meant to have clinicians from different backgrounds share their piece of care, this leads to the risk of no one clinician knowing much about the patient. That is, there is no single clinician who is the primary repository for knowledge about the patient. This can lead to team members pulling in different directions with regard to care without realizing it.

Lack of Staff Training

Many staff have a cursory knowledge of eating disorders if any at all. Trying to educate the whole team to be equally knowledgeable can be a daunting task if not an impossible one. With team members rotating through different shift schedules including those who come off service to fill in shifts, scratching out in-service times for education can be very difficult. It usually ends up that only a few core team members receive some formal training. Education must, however, be delivered by those who are knowledgeable themselves otherwise treatment can be very misdirected.

Avoidance Because of Bad Experiences With Past Treatment

It's not hard to relate to those who have had bad experiences with previous treatment attempts. Assessments should always include questions regarding past treatments. We want to know what worked as well as what didn't seem to work. We also want to know why treatment was successful or why it may not have been.

When an individual says that they didn't like or even hated a particular treatment, ask why. Treatment may have not been what they expected. They may have been expected to achieve something they didn't want to, but actually was a reasonable option such as increasing nutrition intake and possibly weight gain. Other times, there may have been treatment options that were inappropriate or just plain wrong.

The concept of *bad experiences* is open to interpretation by patients, caregivers and family. Sometimes we don't know what is appropriate treatment or what may or may not work until it is tried. There are, however, definite *don't do* treatment options. Regardless of the best intentions of staff, staff attitudes may have been inappropriate or even toxic.

If we see sources of poor treatment, let others know.

Examples of "bad" experiences:

- Expecting nutrition or weight increases when individuals are not ready
- Keeping people in treatment long after recovery goals have not been met and are not likely to be in the near future
- Insisting on treatments that were not agreed upon by staff and individual
- Given inappropriate drugs
- Being treated for an incorrect diagnosis
- Being belittled or blamed
- Any punitive actions
- Being denied contact with significant others when it may have been useful
- Being expected to spend time with family, partners, or other significant others when this could have been harmful
- Being allowed to leave hospital treatment resulting in suicide attempt
- Individuals mixed with others with eating disorders who are trying to undo treatment expectations or are using drugs and alcohol in treatment
- Relationship with caregivers has been sexualized
- Romantic relationships between patients

- Serious attempts by patient to work on recovery but cannot meet goals or lose ground after discharge
- Being accused of splitting when was not
- Changing staff where there were some "good ones" and others that did not seem to care or were punitive
- Drug reactions
- Admitted to religious-based treatment programs and asked "What would Christ do is this situation?"
- Expected to eat foods they do not want to eat such as hot dogs when the individual was a vegetarian prior to the eating disorder
- Unrealistic goals.
- Non-negotiated goals
- Inconsistent treatment. That is, different staff expect different objectives.
- Shifting goals
- Transfer of care to caregivers that they do not connect with or are *on another page* with treatment objectives
- A bad experience may be that someone was in good or appropriate treatment that was discontinued due to the family moving away, returning home before treatment was finished, finances, retirement of therapist, eating disorder program funding cut, treatment ends for an individual in an adolescent program because they have turned 19 and an adult eating disorder program was not readily available
- Experienced acute depression and suicidal ideation or psychosis during treatment for an eating disorder
- Unhoped for weight gain on ward even if expected
- Sexual or physical assault by another patient during admission
- Flashbacks
- Patient became worse during treatment
- Overtly frustrated staff

Lack of Treatment Resources

Adequate treatment resources for those with eating disorders, on the average, are scarce worldwide. Most resources are in major population centers and will be inaccessible for the majority of individuals that require them. These programs may serve a few adequately but for the most part fall short of fulfilling the needs of most. Some of the reasons for this are as follows.

Lack of a Complete Set of Treatment Resources

Although major treatment centers provide a multitude of services, they are never complete. They may provide hospital and or residential care, meal support, nutrition counseling, life skills groups, one-on-one therapist time including access to a psychiatrist, occupational therapist, and various other assorted services. So what's missing?

Most programs are either adult or pediatric. Others may span from late adolescence such as 17 years of age to young adult about 25 years of age. What typically happens with those who have had care in an adolescent program is that they have nowhere else to continue treatment after. Rarely there is a seamless transfer of care to an adult program when the individual becomes too old for the adolescent program. A complete halt to treatment may end there. Even if there may be an adult program available there will likely be a significant wait time for entry. Some wait times may be for months and even over a year due to long waitlists.

Some cities may offer hospital treatment to adults only and not to children or adolescents. As well they may only offer outpatient nutrition counseling for either adolescents or adults but not both.

There is typically an absence of *step-down programs*. Individuals may be a part of a 24/7 hospital or residential program and then they will be discharged to the community where there are either no resources or possibly an hour weekly visit with a counselor or dietitian at best. This allows the return of the stressors and lack of support they experienced prior to admission to the in-depth program.

Bed Availability

When I was initially working in the area of eating disorders, I had to admit clients to any ward in the hospital that would take them. It might be a surgical, medical, gynecological, or any other ward that was available. I have had to admit individuals to an emergency ward for a few days due to bed shortages. My dream was to have a single ward dedicated to treating those with eating disorders for logistical reasons and to have the availability of a trained ward staff knowledgeable about eating disorder management. Regarding logistics, I admitted to two hospitals miles apart and one pediatric psychiatric facility. I spent as much time driving between the centers as providing clinical services. That day did come when there was one and only one place dedicated to eating disorder treatment for adults. What this did was to shut down access for admission to all other wards and patients had to be on a waitlist in the only two designated eating disorder ward beds. At least by having individuals admitted to different ward services, some degree of safety, especially for those with significant medical and suicide risks, could be provided on the interim until a bed was available on the eating disorder ward.

Lack of Skilled Clinicians

Very few clinicians have any adequate training in the field of eating disorders. Even if they have had some training, it will not have been nearly enough. Some treatment programs who offer eating disorder management recruit therapists who are willing to learn on-the-run, as it were, while on the job.

Treatment Programs Too Far Away

Some major treatment programs offer an outpatient day program out of a hospital. This is fine for those who live in town but will make access unrealistic for others. One would have to be able to afford rent for an apartment in the city with the program.

Lack of Financial Resources

Some individuals and families will have insurance coverage for treatment of eating disorders but many will not. Even if there are accessible programs many cannot afford them. With hospital and residential programs costing $2000 a day or more, few have this kind of money. Even weekly counseling sessions can cost hundreds of dollars per visit. As eating disorders are chronic conditions, a month or two of treatment is not likely to be enough. Treatment sometimes needs to continue for months if not years.

Revolving Door

With the deficiencies of programs, there is a *revolving door* access to treatment for many. Some will get the extra time they need for treatment by reentering programs several times if this is, indeed, possible. With some requiring repeated treatment, this takes away treatment time for others who need it. In turn, this increases waitlist times. Some actively seek repeated treatment because programs are the only social connections they have. Remaining ill is a benefit to them.

Falling Between the Cracks

One of the greatest contributors to failed treatment attempts are when individuals, families as well as caregivers fall between the cracks of any number of systems or agencies. These may include hospital, insurance, government, social services, police, drug and alcohol, sexual assault, and multiple other medical and mental health services. Non-profit support groups such as Alcoholics Anonymous, Narcotics Anonymous, and those for eating disorders, sexual assault, violence against women, and so on may become useful. These services are often in short supply. Even if these services are accessible, the timing of appointments or group participation may be unrealistic for those wishing to utilize them. Employment, school, or medical appointments may conflict.

Some of the reasons individuals and families fall between the cracks are:

- Many of the needed agencies required do no exist in the community. They may only exist in larger populations.
- Many agencies or treatment facilities have long waitlists.
- Funding for treatment programs get cut.
- Coordination for access to treatment options or other services is impossible
- Seamless transfer of services is not built into health systems. That is, each service functions alone and not in an integrated fashion.
- Transfer from child and adolescent facilities to an adult facility is not possible. This may be because the adult treatment center is in another city as well as there is no coordinated transfer of care planning.
- Referral letters were not written
- Parents pull their children from current treatment in favor of another. Alternative or fad treatment options become favored. It's hard to be too critical of families that chose these other options when so-called evidence-based methods fail and individuals or families have already lost a fortune.
- People don't show for appointments and have to rebook. A new referral letter may have to be written.
- Changing program administrations may result in changes in admission criteria and treatment protocols.
- Specialists refuse to rebook individuals who keep canceling, do not show for appointments or do not follow treatment recommendations
- Clinicians cancel appointments and individuals need to rebook.
- Entry criteria for treatment programs may be too strict.
- Individuals become ill with a different condition that needs immediate attention and, therefore, requires putting off eating disorder and other services already being lined up. The new or more dominant health issue such as severe chronic pain, drug and alcohol addiction, or advancing multiple sclerosis comes front and center. A single relatively simple surgical procedure such as having a gallbladder removed can cause a chain reaction of resource accesses coming undone. In many cases, arranging treatment resources becomes like a game of Snakes and Ladders where when one loses their place in line for a particular treatment, they have to go back to the very beginning and start all over.
- Individuals become lost to follow-up due to substance abuse, getting a job, or going to college as well as having given up on the idea that treatment will work. They may have just moved away and dropped all contact with treatment programs, family, and friends.
- Suicide prevention programs were not utilized.

Repeated Failure of Treatments

With the best efforts of patients, families, and caregivers, treatment efforts may fail or at least seem to fail in the short term. Repeated treatment efforts that continue to not meet recovery goals bring further frustration to all involved. Where the financial costs of treatment has to be born by families or individuals, repeated failed treatments can be met with massive debts and nothing to show for it. Months, years and sometimes decades of failed treatment attempts are spirit and heartbreaking. The whole process becomes completely demoralizing. Trying to persuade someone to work on recovery yet again when all previous attempts have failed can be sheer torture for individuals, their family or partner. It becomes a "Here we go again" scenario.

Ward culture

Hospital and residential treatment wards for those with eating disorders provide structure, emotional support, and a directed treatment path. For the most part, this is a positive and necessary platform for recovery. The issue is that wards can be rife with complicating and destructive forces.

Drug and Alcohol Use

A significant other concern on wards is the use of drugs and alcohol. Though treatment programs diligently screen for active substance use, the process falls very short of being effective. Some programs provide various groups for inpatients and outpatients. These groups can be designed for nutrition education, yoga, self-esteem, and others. The concern is that many groups allow water bottles. Some bottles will be in of the Thermos type or clear plastic. It has been reported that all individuals in various groups will fill the bottles with vodka or gin and facilitators are none to the wiser. Substance use during treatment for an eating disorder really is an indication of a total lack of willingness to engage in recovery efforts. This behavior takes away the opportunity for those who could truly benefit from the program but instead have to remain on a waitlist.

Negative Eating Disorder Culture and Contamination Amongst Patients

During my training as an intern at the city hospital, I witnessed destructive influences of eating disorder ward culture. Instead of individuals in treatment dedicating to their own recovery, they would deliberately undo treatment objectives by any means possible. Some of these methods of undoing are as follows.

- Clients would drink fluids, tape cutlery to themselves or stuff a bottle of shampoo into their underwear before being weighed.
- Running up and down stairs during passes to burn calories
- Throwing food out as well as vomiting meals and snacks
- Exercising under their bed covers
- Laxatives, suppositories, emetics, or Gravol would be smuggled in by friends or purchased from pharmacies while out on passes.
- Friends would smuggle in drugs and alcohol
- Falsely claim they have food allergies, gluten intolerance, or are vegetarians

A common trend is that clients share eating disorder secrets in order to help others engage more successfully in meeting eating disorder goals including further weight loss. Clients would contaminate others on the ward with their toxic weight loss agenda. It was a misery loves company kind of scenario. It's not unlike those who go to prison who learn prison culture and leave with more engrained criminal attitudes and skills. Those that enter hospital or residential eating disorder treatment programs can be discharged with worse eating disorder attitudes and more destructive behaviors. When a patient enters a program having lost 20 lbs and meets someone who had lost 75 lbs, the weight loss bar has then been lowered to an extreme. Patients may conclude that they originally had wimpy weight loss goals prior to admission and now must meet a new standard.

How Can Experts Make Mistakes?

Regardless of how well educated, up-to-date or experienced clinically we are, we will make mistakes, even those that can be lethal. With our best efforts, sometimes we zig when we should zag. "To err is human …"

Some examples of colossal blunders by highly intelligent, highly accomplished and highly decorated individual or teams are as follows.

The Hubble telescope was sent into orbit in 1990. It was to be the most powerful telescope in space designed to unlock secrets of the universe. When scientists first tested it in space they discovered that it would not focus. Oops!. There was a miniscule spherical aberration in the manufacturing of the main mirror. Fortunately the telescope was built with the possibility of repairs in mind. It was the first space telescope to be repairable – a fortunate bit of insight. NASA had to send a repair team into space and added a device with ten small mirrors to correct the problem. Routine maintenance or *preventive maintenance* missions were then organized. A total of five repair missions were needed eventually. How can a team of brilliant physicists, mathematicians, and engineers have missed that the telescope would not focus before launch? It happens.

During the second gulf war, the US military bragged that they could not only hit a specific building in a war zone but could send a missile into any given window of a building. Their computer guided missiles were that accurate, at least they thought. News came out during the war that these warheads were hitting hospitals and schools. This should not have been able to happen but it did.

Stories of medical errors abound. The classic blunder is when a surgeon amputates the wrong leg. The anesthetist as well as nurses involved in the surgery all are aware of the designated leg to be removed but also fail to thwart the demise.

In summary, we are all going to make mistakes, but being as prepared as we can be and attempting to anticipate risk will aid us in diminishing error.

Gut Feelings. Trust Them or Not?

Gut feelings are just that – feelings or hunches. Do we trust them or not? The best advise I can give is to pay attention to them and act on the ones that could help anticipate a real crisis in evolution.

A couple of times I have had a hunch that a particular teenage patient was going to attempt suicide. Once when I visited her at the pediatric psychiatric facility she was sitting outside on a nice sunny day with a grin on her face. I interpreted this to mean that she was up to something and I confronted her. I said "Are you planning to kill yourself?" She fessed up that she had already taken 100 tablets of acetaminophen. Needless to say, she was taken to the emergency room for treatment after which she survived. Another time, she was visiting the pediatric ward in the general hospital, she had been admitted to a few times previously. I asked her why she was there. She said that she was just riding around on her bike visiting the staff on this ward after having visited staff at the psychiatric facility. I said to her, "You're not saying hello, your saying goodbye. You're going to kill yourself aren't you?" Her face dropped and she then ran off the ward and went down the stairs to escape the hospital. I phoned security and they caught her trying to leave the hospital. If I had not visited just at the exact moment she had taken the overdose at the psychiatric hospital or had been visiting the general pediatric ward when she was there, she may have lost her life. Having said this, we cannot really know what would ultimately have happened.

Another time, I was visiting patients on an adult psychiatric unit and a patient walked by the nursing unit where I was writing a note and she said "Dr. Kirkpatrick. I just want to let you know how much I appreciate everything you have done for me." I thanked her. I then took a moment to consider that this was an inappropriate statement made for no obvious reason. I spoke to her nurse and said "I think she is going to kill herself." The nurse went to her room and found her trying to hang herself in the shower." If she had not spoken to me, she might have died. This attempt was serious. It was only by chance that I was on that ward at just that moment. I could have easily done rounds earlier or later that day.

There are other times when I had not sensed suicidal ideation and some have followed through with a suicide and others have attempted but lived. Error on the side of caution regardless. We may have gut feelings with regard to medical demise as well. Act on these too. If we are wrong, then no harm done.

Anticipating Medical Crises in Eating Disorders. Really?

Anticipating any event depends on many factors. Some anticipations are certainties such as expecting the sun will rise tomorrow while others are extremely remote events such as an asteroid colliding with earth. Anticipating that critical events will actually happen and when for those with eating disorders is somewhere in between these two extremes. How many clinicians have worried for months and sometimes years over whether their client will drop dead but it has never happened, at least to date. How many times have we not worried so much or were, indeed, not aware of serious risks and then a client experiences serious health events or even death. The best any of us can do is to be as alert as possible and put our supportive ducks in a row. We are not trying to anticipate when or where a specific crisis will happen but that it *can* happen and is at the front of our mind.

A number of non-healthcare professionals build *anticipation* into their work life. Some examples of this are as follows.

The iconic hockey player, Wayne Gretsky, who has won six Stanley Cups and an Olympic gold medal is famous for saying "I skate to where the puck is going to be, not to where it has been." A significant issue for those who treat eating disorders is that we likely do not have a vision of where eating disorder treatment is going to go for any given person. We can, however, be aware of the *possibilities* of where the eating disorder may lead and plan for these as best as we can.

Airplane pilots always determine the expected weather before taking flight. They anticipate that weather can change and want to be prepared for untoward and dangerous changes. The same is true for spaceship launches. Even if the current weather is adequate for launch, cautions are taken for possible weather changes that may evolve the following day or even hours before launch. Launches may be canceled or delayed over the most minor of risks.

Farmers are often plagued with not knowing long-term or even short-term weather outcomes. The possibility of too much or too little rain, too much or too little sunshine as well as it could be too cold or too hot are anticipated. Grasshopper and caterpillar infestations are also on the minds of farmers. There is no crystal ball for predicting weather or pest threats but knowing ahead of time they may happen, farmers may build in some preparation and safeguards. Mental readiness may be our best defense.

When in medical school I had an interest in neurosurgery. So I did several elective rotations with the chief of neurosurgery who took me under his wing. I mentored under his resident as well. One day the chief said "Come with me. We're going to attend an operation that has gone terribly wrong. When you go in, stand at the patient's head by the anesthetist and don't say a thing." What had happened was that the operating surgeon was an orthopedic surgeon and was performing neck surgery. The patient was face down on the table and the spine of the neck was exposed from above. The surgeon had inadvertently drilled through the vertebral artery on the left side. Blood was everywhere. He had called my supervisor to help him save the patient's life. He said to the anesthetist to hang a bag of Nipride, sodium nitroprusside, to lower the blood pressure to a systolic reading of 90. The surgeon then took a flap of adjacent neck muscle and sewed it over the ruptured artery as had been advised him. This saved the day.

This event occurred in the era when orthopedic surgeons were the new kids on the block with regard to performing spinal surgery. They were the hotshots of the operating room and had the newest and spiffiest surgical tools of the day. The neurosurgeons were seen somewhat as a bunch of fuddy-duddies doing things "the old way". What the orthopedic surgeons did not do ahead of surgery was order four pints of cross-matched blood. The neurosurgeons always did before performing neck surgery. They anticipated a worse case scenario should it actually occur. This undoubtedly developed from years of neck surgery experience having learned the hard way cross-matched blood was essential. Some surgeons and other medical practitioners are so sure of their skills that they believe they could never possibly make such a serious error as described above.

I consulted with my supervisor after and said "It must be nice to know that your chances of making a serious error are almost non-existent given your decade or so of excellent results." He said "I fully anticipate that I can still make a catastrophic error. A surgeon needs to know all of the things that can go wrong and be prepared when they happen." The neurosurgeons may have been old-school but their wisdom paid off here. This brings to mind cliché sayings such as the boy scout motto: "Be Prepared" and "Expect the worst and hope for the best."

Redundancy and Preventive Maintenance

Two words should be engrained into the minds of healthcare workers and providers. They are **redundancy** and **preventive maintenance.**

Redundancy

In the medical world we tend to use the words *backup treatment* or *options we can fall back on* in place of redundancy. Often, however, these back-up or fall back options are often seen as *afterthoughts* or "We'll figure it out later if things don't work out." How many times have we chosen a treatment option, hoping it might work, and end up left with no viable alternatives when treatment really doesn't end up working as expected. The back-up plans we were hoping for were actually not available, at least when we needed them. Or possibly, the back-up options were too expensive for families and individuals or resources were too far away in another city. In healthcare, hoped for back-up options are all too often loosey-goosey. We don't seem to realize this until we actually need a plan B right now. In areas of science, redundancy is hardwired into research and development. In the aerospace industry, redundancy is the norm and pretty much a sacred quest.

Whether talking about airliners, fighter jets, rockets, satellites, Mars rovers, or space stations, redundancy is everything. Although scientists are not able to have redundancy for everything that could go wrong, they work hard to provide it especially for the more essential functions of machines.

When preparing the care for those with eating disorders, put into place as many Plan Bs as possible.

These Plan Bs may be to:

- Having a reliable colleague or two willing to cover for you when you are not available for designated times off such as evenings or weekends and also for unexpected times you may be absent such as illness, family emergencies, or you happen to miss your plane flight. Make sure your colleagues are familiar with your care plan and, if possible, introduce them to your patient ahead of time.
- Have all contact information of family, partners and supportive services yourself and also of others that share the management of ones care. Should a client disappear from a ward or their home, make sure all loved ones and caregivers can contact each other without your involvement in order to provide an effective network to aid in locating the individual.
- Make sure all caregivers on a ward or in a treatment program are familiar with the treatment goals and know how to contact each other should you not be available.
- Have a critical emergency medical treatment plan in place should ones medical status escalate whether in the community or in a hospital setting.

Preventive Maintenance

My father was an engineer for the Royal Canadian Air Force. When I was about ten years old I asked him what he did in his work, he said that he was responsible for the *preventive maintenance* of large mechanical devices on the airbase. This included the functioning of the jetfighter alert hangers where jets with nuclear tipped missiles could be scrambled in the air under two minutes. The twelve hanger door motors all had to work perfectly in unison in order to lift the doors that weighed several tons and perform this quickly. He was also responsible for ground approach radar installations as well as their maintenance.

What preventive maintenance was about was making sure mechanical things were inspected routinely while trouble shooting for early disrepair and then fixing them before a major breakdown occurred. Benjamin Franklin once said "An ounce of prevention is worth a pound of cure" with regard to preventing fires in Philadelphia. Clinicians can save themselves and others a lot of misery by anticipating events, when possible, that could go awry and preparing for them ahead of time.

Chapter 2

Stories of Critical and Lethal Medical Scenarios

Stories of Critical and Lethal Medical Scenarios help to imitate the experience of real-life clinical situations. This is a task not possible by attempting to piecemeal didactic medical or psychological text.

The *Stories* cover a vast array of clinical possibilities. Some may start out presenting seemingly minimal clinical indicators but then evolve to reveal critical or even lethal outcomes. Other *Stories* relay critical medical scenarios up-front resolving to positive outcomes or possibly death. A few do not purvey crisis, per say, but deliver a message of importance, in other words, "pay attention."

Some *Stories* quote statements from autopsy and coroner's reports. The coroner's comments provide the most stirring and emotionally grounding information. The core purpose of our work with those with eating disorders can be felt here.

Most *Stories* are a composite of lived events, thus, commanding our most sincere reverence.

Angel's Story

Angel was a 34 year-old university professor. She emigrated from Ireland with her parents when she was 3 years old. Her story highlights the plethora of eating disorder behaviors one can be engaged in. She was 5'4', 98 lbs with a BMI of 16.3 when she first came for treatment of her eating disorder. Her weight had been as low as 78 lbs, a BMI of 13.4 a year earlier.

Her eating disorder behaviors included:

• Restricting food intake from between 400 to 900 calories daily on average.
• Some days she would drink only water.
• She would weigh herself 5 to15 times per day with 10 being the average. She weighed herself first thing in the morning after voiding. She then weighed herself after eating, exercising, vomiting, and after bowel movements.

DOI: 10.4324/9781003053088-2

- Angel vomited multiple times daily.
- She wore tight fitting trousers and shirts to help gauge changes in body shape as a reflection of weight changes.
- She looked into the mirror whenever possible throughout the day.
- She would eat using toy doll cutlery including a knife, fork, and spoon.
- She secretly spit food into a napkin or into a drinking cup when eating at the dinner table with her family. She disposed food in the napkin or cup after dinner. She ate with family only when she could not avoid it.
- She threw food away after she hoarded food for some time in her bedroom.
- She would purchase tampons so family would think she was having periods even though she experienced amenorrhea for over a year.
- She refused to eat with others at work and would only eat a small salad for lunch if at all.
- She cut food into small pieces in order to slow eating down as this would allow time for a full feeling to develop before she felt she ate too much.
- She walked three to five hours most days.
- She vomited until she saw either bile or blood during sessions of vomiting
- She would fluid load with water during vomiting sessions to liquefy food thus making vomiting easier. She drank water after vomiting each individual time until she vomited clear water only, indicating to her she had removed all food from her stomach.
- She stopped vomiting if she experienced chest pain because of fear of doing serious harm to herself such as tearing her stomach or esophagus possibly resulting in death.

Because she experienced palpitations, she required a cardiac investigation. Testing included EKGs, an echocardiogram, Holter monitor as well as an event monitor. She also had an extensive hematological workup and urinalysis. It was discovered that she had a severe metabolic alkylosis and hypomagnesemia.

She was contacted by the cardiac monitoring center that had been observing her cardiac electrical patterns in real-time while she wore a Holter monitor. They told her to go to the emergency room stat due to a life-threatening tracing. She was admitted to the intensive care units (ICU) with a *torsades de pointes* cardiac dysrhythmia – a precursor to sudden cardiac death.

When initially admitted to ICU one clinician asked her how many times a day had she been vomiting. She told her that she vomited 4 times daily. The very next day, another clinician asked the same question. "How many times a day have you been vomiting?" She said "I vomit 20 times, 4 times a day." That is she had been vomiting 80 times daily and even more. Reworded, she was vomiting 20 times during each of 4 sessions of vomiting most days.

When asked how many *sessions* of vomiting she may carry out in a day she said there could be between 2 and 6 sessions daily during which she may attempt vomiting 5 to 25 times each session.

Angel and her sister were getting ready to go to bed when Angel fell to the ground unresponsive. Paramedics were called and they pronounced Angel dead upon arrival. The paramedics discovered bags of potassium and magnesium supplements in her bedroom that had been prescribed by her family doctor, but obviously had not been taken.

Discussion

There were a number of events that set the stage for a lethal outcome. However, a number of positive steps had been taken by Angel in conjunction with her family doctor that could have saved the day. What went wrong?

She engaged in over fifteen eating disorder related behaviors. Some of them were very dangerous such as daily extensive vomiting sessions. Severe restricting would also have contributed to risk of life threatening metabolic disorders.

Angel went through the motions of appropriate medical monitoring from time to time. She visited her doctor, had vital signs taken, and was weighed. She took the lab requisition provided by her doctor for extensive hematological and urine screening. She went to the laboratory and had the screening done. When the critical lab results arrived at her doctor's office, she would make an appointment with her and showed up for review of results. She accepted the prescriptions for magnesium and potassium supplement and had them filled. The supplements made it home. What is missing is that she did not take her supplements and essentially hoarded them. Could her family doctor have done more? The only thing possibly that could have been done, if it had not already been so, was that she could have insisted on laboratory blood testing on a daily basis by phoning Angel daily. After receiving the results of the reports, the doctor could then recommend medication adjustments until improved results appeared. If lab reports were not improving or even getting worse, it should have been insisted that Angel go to the hospital for medical stabilization. A *medical treatment loop* – a complete chain of treatment options linked without a single step being overlooked – needs to be put in place, when possible, for everyone requiring medical management.

The three EKG tracings shown at the beginning of *Preface* are those of Angel's. They were recorded as the paramedics were performing an unsuccessful resuscitation.

Lesson Points

- Regardless of how thorough medical investigations seem to be, make sure the *medical treatment loop* is being carried out with very close patient contact. In other words, nag more! If possible, admit those with critical medical risks to hospital until there is a safe degree of stabilization and replacement of nutrients.

Erica's Story

I was contacted by a cardiologist requesting an eating disorder consultation for Erica who had lost 40 lbs in eleven months but denied having an eating disorder. She was admitted to the cardiac ward with a history of palpitations, some dizziness and chest pains but did not have a history of syncope, loss of consciousness or shortness of breath. Erica was 28 years old, 5'6", 106 lbs and had a BMI of 17.1. The cardiologist said he wanted me to see her by noon as he was going to discharge her immediately after. Considering I couldn't get to the hospital untill after noon, this became quite a challenge. Having been engrained in my clinical behavior from medical school that we as physicians should read the chart *first* before seeing the patient in person, this is exactly what I did. The following is what I saw when I opened the file (Figures 2.1–2.10).

I immediately became aware of the plethora of various abnormal electro-cardiograph tracings. Note the various EKG tracing interpretations during a single visit to the cardiac ward.

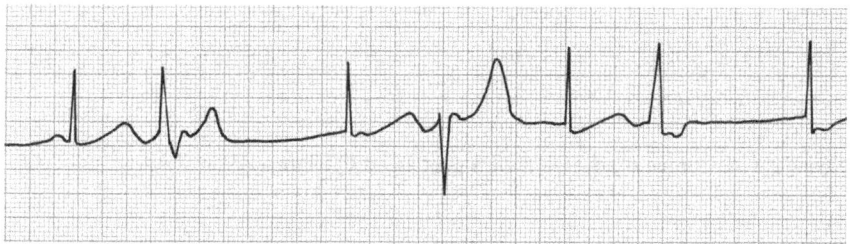

Figure 2.1 Junctional rhythm punctuated by polymorphic PVCs.

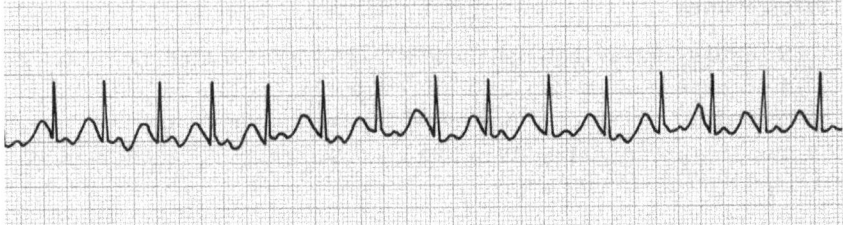

Figure 2.2 Narrow complex tachycardia or SVT.

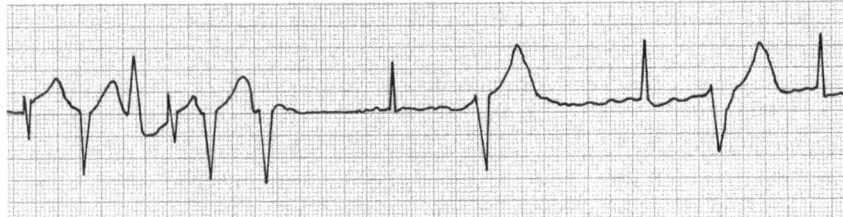

Figure 2.3 5 beat polymorphic ventricular tachycardia followed by period of ventricular bigeminy.

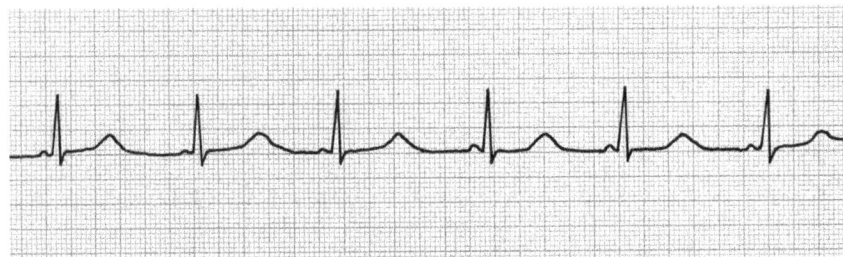

Figure 2.4 Junctional bradycardia with prolonged QT interval.

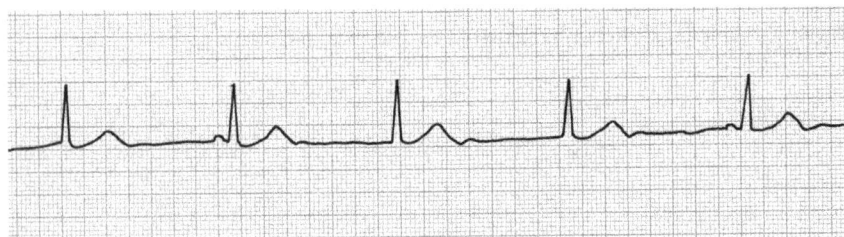

Figure 2.5 Junctional bradycardia.

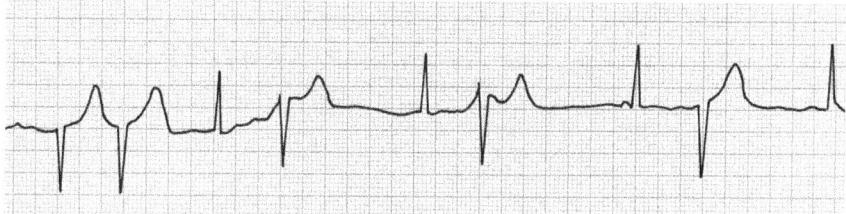

Figure 2.6 Junctional bradycardia with frequent monomorphic PVCs.

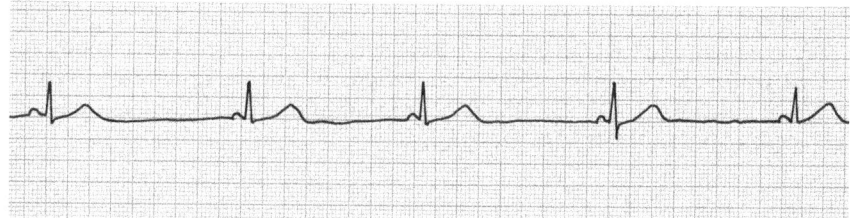

Figure 2.7 Junctional bradycardia.

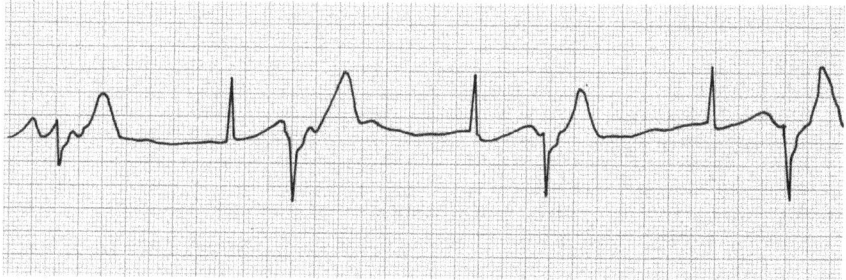

Figure 2.8 Junctional bradycardia with ventricular bigeminy.

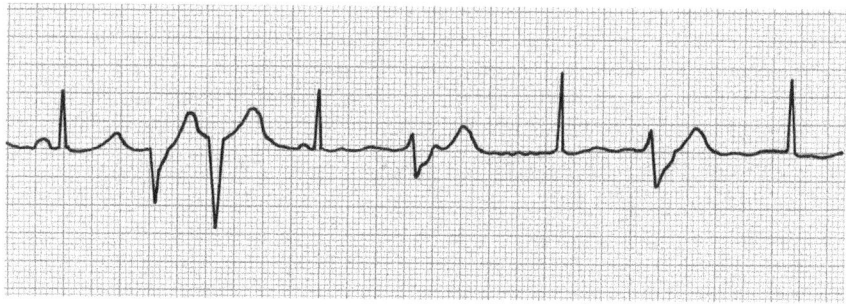

Figure 2.9 Junctional rhythm with polymorphic PVCs.

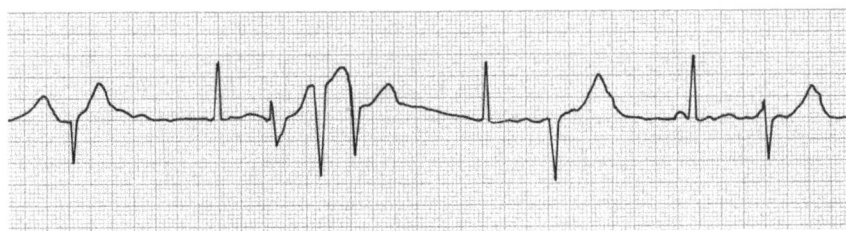

Figure 2.10 Junctional rhythm with polymorphic PVCs including one ventricular triplet.

After noting the EKG tracings I then came across the Holter monitor report. Notice the stunning number and kinds of abnormal cardiac events reported. Out of over almost 75,000 QRS complexes recorded, just under 10,000 were abnormal. That's approximately 14% that were abnormal.

Holter monitor report

9580 isolated ventricular ectopic beats were reported and of these there were:

- 9251 bigeminal cycles
- 219 couplets
- 27 runs
- 73 beats in runs
- 6 beats at 133 bpm
- 4 beats at 156 bpm

The lowest heart rate reported was 28 bpm.

Of all the EKG tracings that I reviewed the most benign looking one, if it was to be seen at a glance, was the one with the most lethality associated with it. This was a 12 lead EKG. The student in training or a physician distracted during a hectic day could miss its ominous message. This tracing showed normal QRS and p wave complexes. No extra or absent beats appeared. There was no evidence of ischemia either. The HR was reported as 52 bpm which is just a bit bradycardic. What was ominous about this tracing was the *prolonged QTc interval* of 625 msec. This can be a harbinger for sudden cardiac death. Although the previous several tracings are far more eye catching and would bring trepidation to many clinicians, this last one is one of the bad ones for which we need to have an acute awareness.

The echocardiogram report revealed more insight into a yet more compounding clinical story. Of note, it stated "mild to moderate mitral valve leaflet prolapse affecting both leaflets. No insufficiency was detected."

Hospital standard vitals record sheets are designed to allow staff to record the most extreme of vital activities for the most ill and even dying patients. In this instance, the nurse recorded below the allotted charting area for temperature. Erica's temperature went as low as 35.8 C (96.4 F) with the highest being 37.4 C (99.3 F) over a five day period. The temperature rose from the lowest in this record to a 1.2 C (2.2 F) jump in one day. The temperature also varied within half of a degree in a two-hour period. This is a very abnormal temperature recording. Whether the core temperature of an individual is recorded at the north-pole or at the equator, it remains the same in the healthy person. This temperature record is indicative of *autonomic dysfunction*, a serious indicator of potential demise. The hospital record also showed that the blood pressure was varied greatly and went as low as 64 over 40 at one point. Aside from multiple dysrhythmias, Erica was hypomagnesemic as well as hypoglycemia upon admission.

After reviewing the chart, I then introduced myself to Erica and acquired a history from her. Below are highlights of her medical history gleaned from our initial assessment as well as from subsequent assorted consultant reports. Because data was collected from multiple sources, the timeline for events listed is not necessarily precise.

- Erica had a diagnosis of mitral valve prolapse at 11 years old and hypercholesterolemia soon after. A specialist's report stated that she had "lax ligaments."
- Her father died young at 51 years of age from a myocardial infarction when Erica was 12 years old.
- She was put on a restricting diet by her family doctor at 15 years-old because of familial hypercholesterolemia. She weighed 140 lbs at the time.
- She became conscious of her weight at 13 years old.
- She began the Jenny Craig diet in grade 12 so she could lose weight for health reasons and not because she felt overweight.
- She had an overall restricting history of 5 years.
- In high school, she worked at a restaurant where girls were talking about dieting and their dissatisfaction with their own weight.
- She lost from 154 lbs to 106 lbs over a two-year period. She had lost 44 lbs over the previous 11 months. Her clothing size went from 10 to 4.
- There was no history of binging, vomiting, over exercising, or Ipecac use. Nor had there been any other eating disorder behaviors reported.
- Erica had a hard time accepting that she had an eating disorder as she truly felt her dieting and weight changes had nothing to do with body image control.

- An Eating Disorder Inventory (EDI) had been done, at the tertiary care eating disorder program where she had been admitted, showing a 3%ile body dissatisfaction score. That is, she had almost no body image dissatisfaction.
- One consultant's note stated that the physical exam revealed a Grade II/VI late systolic murmur and temperature of 36.2 C (97.2 F). Her BP was 70/50 that visit.
- Her general medical history identified that she experienced migraine headaches and was taking cisipride, an intestinal dysmotility modifier. Because cisipride was becoming known for being associated with sudden cardiac death in a number of those with anorexia nervosa, I discontinued the prescription for this.

Erica ended up seeing four cardiologists in two cities and a medical specialist in eating disorders in the tertiary care eating disorder program. After treatment at the hospital and with myself, she was able to gain weight. Her cardiac status improved to the point where her EKGs were normal and a cardiologist described her cardiac status as "benign." She did not require any cardioactive medications, pacemaker, or defibrillator as had been considered.

After recovery, she admitted she wanted to lose weight after all. She said she did not realize this at the time and I believed her.

Coroner's Comments

SUMMARY OF EVENTS

"Erica G. was kissing her boyfriend goodnight when she suddenly collapsed. The ambulance service arrived within 1–2 minutes and found her to be in atrial fibrillation. They commenced full cardiac protocols and were able to find some electrical activity after administering atropine, however there was never any output. She was transferred to the hospital and shortly after arrival, death was pronounced by the emergency room physician.

MEDICAL HISTORY

As a child it was reported that she had a heart murmur and then no other problems until a few years later. At that time she had lost 30 lbs and had missed three menstrual cycles after stopping the oral contraceptive pill. She also had a very low heart rate with runs of ventricular ectopy, mitral valve prolapse, and lax ligaments. She also suffered from familial hypercholesterolemia and near blackouts and palpitations daily. She later had a number of hospitalizations relating to these problems. There were also concerns regarding eating disorders, these were not clinically proven.

POST MORTEM AND TOXICOLOGICAL EXAMINATIONS

The post mortem confirmed the mitral valve prolapse as well as cardiomegaly and focal atherosclerosis of the right anterior descending and circumflex arteries. It also confirmed a slight myxoid deposition at annular attachment. Toxicology screen was negative.

CONCLUSIONS

This inquiry finds that Ms. G. died of a cardiac arrhythmia due to a floppy mitral valve with prolapse.

I classify this death as natural."

Discussion

Erica presented with low weight, palpitations, and a number of abnormal EKG tracings. She was hypokalemic, hypomagnesemic as well as hypoglycemic. I assumed her medical status was critical although almost all of the EKG tracings were not necessarily a threat and the hypomagnesemia as well as hypoglycemia were not extreme. I was worried about medical risks not yet identified such as more serious EKG patterns emerging or the worsening of existing abnormal laboratory results.

After what seemed remarkable recovery with regard to nutrition, weight, cardiac status, and laboratory values, Erica died regardless. Underlying her previously serious health concerns, she had atherosclerosis and myxoid deposition at annular attachment not identified until autopsy. These findings along with an MVP were likely responsible for the array of abnormal EKG tracings. Starvation with associated metabolic abnormalities likely aggravated the occult aberrant electrical cardiac function. Others with eating disorders having similar medical compromise but without having an MVP and associated electrical conductivity issues would not typically have such electrocardiac irregularities. Her lethal cardiac status was possibly genetically transmitted from her father.

Even after normalization of weight, nutrition, and medical investigations, I was not comfortable with a "benign cardiac" assessment. Erica had been investigated several times by various experts yet the lethality of her health concerns was missed.

Lesson Points

- Be suspicious of atypical expressions of medical compromise as there may be a not-yet-identified etiology for signs, symptoms, and abnormal medical investigation reports.
- Keep suspicions high for risk regardless of the minimizing opinions of others.

Maryanna's Story

Maryanna was 22 years old when I first met her. She would binge eat consuming between 50,000 to 80,000 calories daily as well as would vomit between 20, 30, and 40 times daily or more. She was always hypokalemic and usually hypomagnesemic as well as was in chronic renal failure. She worked two full-time jobs spending one pay cheque on food. Maryanna was found unconscious twice downtown then taken to the hospital where she was admitted to the CICU. It was assumed she developed a dysrhythmia while downtown that could not sustain consciousness. The cardiologist read her the riot act each visit stating that she was going to die if she did not stop the eating disorder. These words did not have any impact on her attitudes toward weight control or her very dangerous behaviors. It is possible she had become numb to the words "You're going to die" because she had heard this from me repeatedly for over a decade. Each time I told her she could die, she would often respond with "But I feel fine." Even with showing her critical lab values and ominous EKG tracings, she would continue undeterred.

Maryanna would usually not go for lab work without me first phoning her and saying that I hadn't seen any lab reports recently. I had made a deal with her that if her potassium level had been less than 2.4 mmol/L, I would insist she go to the emergency room (ER) for treatment. If she refused, I would then tell her I would need to call the police or ambulance service and have her involuntarily taken to the ER. She would, however, end up there on her own, have her blood normalized and be released after about 12 hours. While in the community, if her potassium was 2.4 mmol/L or greater she would not be nagged to go to the hospital. At this potassium level, her heart pattern was normal aside from being a bit bradycardic. Her QTc would be normal. As well, she did not experience palpitations, shortness of breath, loss of consciousness, or chest pain as she might have with more critical lab values. Renal failure would be minimal as well and did not pose an immediate threat.

When she tried to avoid going to the ER, as I suggested, the response would be "I don't want to burden the other workers or let down my boss." This was true people pleasing attitude on her part. I do think, however, that the real reason she would actually go to the ER when I had suggested, was that she did not want to be embarrassed by having the police or paramedics meet her at work and insist she go with them.

Following are a couple of samples of typical laboratory findings and an EKG report that would be acquired during a visit to the ER (Figures 2.11, 2.12 and 2.13).

```
= ELECTROLYTES/RENAL FUNCTION ==========================
```

Na	K	Cl	BICARB	ION GAP	UREA	CREAT
135-145	3.5-5.0	101-111	24-32	0-11	3-7.5	50-100
mmol/L	mmol/L	mmol/L	mmol/L	mmol/L	mmol/L	umol/L

139	4.0	110	27	2	1.0 L	80
	3.4 L					
139	2.8 L	101	31	7	1.0 L	100
	3.1 L					
132 L	1.9 C	93 L	29	10	0.5 L	100

```
COMMENT #1
```

```
CHECKED
```

```
OSMOLALITY
280-300
mmol/kg
```

Figure 2.11 Critically low serum potassium, low chloride and creatinine at the high end of normal: corrected in ER.

```
GLUC-random
3.9-11.0
mmol/L
```

```
4.8
5.6
```

```
== ELECTROLYTES/RENAL FUNCTION ========================
```

Na	K	Cl	BICARB	ION GAP	UREA	CREAT
135-145	3.5-5.0	101-111	24-32	0-11	3-7.5	60-110
mmol/L	mmol/L	mmol/L	mmol/L	mmol/L	mmol/L	umol/L

134 L	2.5 C	86 L	34 H	14 H	3.0	100
135	2.0 C	82 L	38 H	15 H	4.0	120 H

```
COMMENT #1
```

```
CHECKED
```

```
= PROTEINS/MINERALS/URIC ACID ========================
```

PROTEIN	ALBUMIN	CALCIUM	MAGNESIUM
63-77	38-53	2.12-2.62	0.70-1.00
g/L	g/L	mmol/L	mmol/L

67	43	2.42	0.88
			0.96

Figure 2.12 Critically low serum K+, low Cl, and elevated bicarb (metabolic alkylosis) and high creatinine. Normal magnesium.

Aside from Maryanna having critical laboratory values, including severe hypokalemia and often metabolic alkylosis, she was almost always in chronic renal failure. The creatinine values reported here as 100 and 120 umol/L are lower than on the average for her. It was not uncommon to see creatinine levels of 140 umol/L or higher on and off for over two decades.

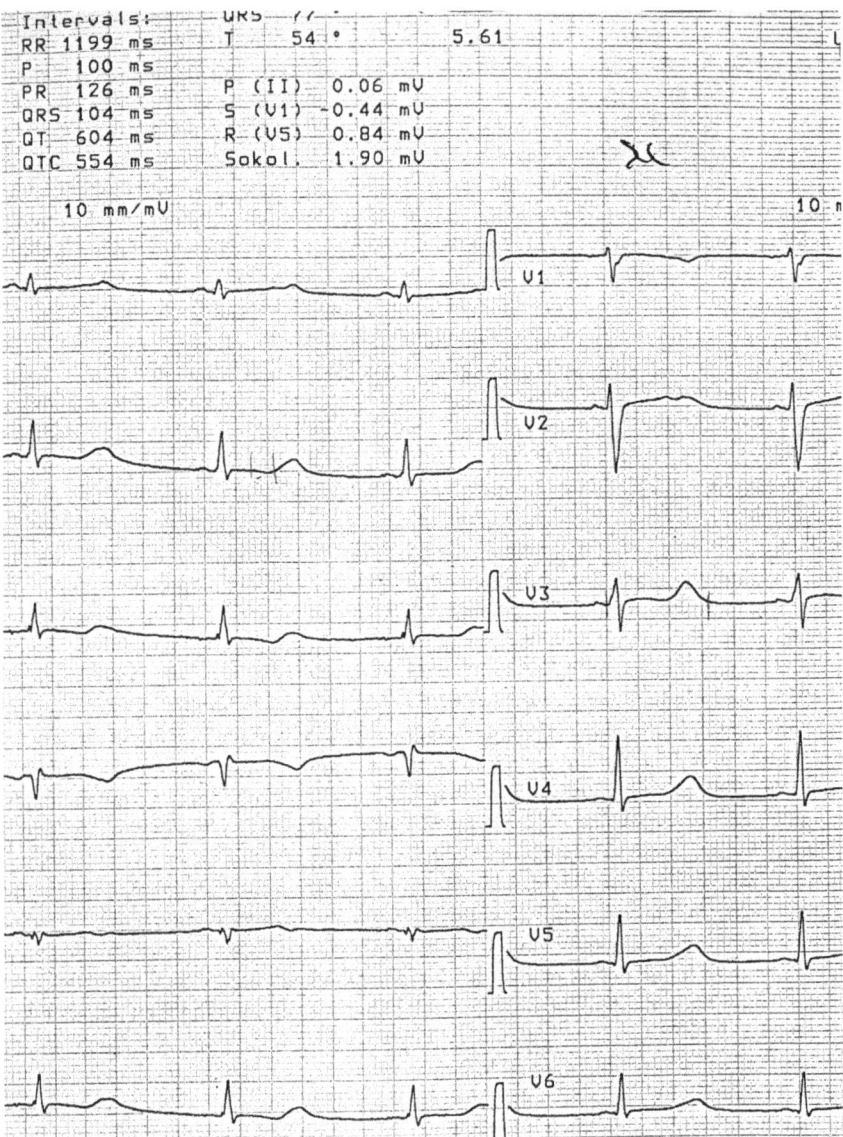

Figure 2.13 12 lead EKG tracing displaying profound QT interval prolongation with mild bradycardia.

This EKG tracing should be seen as a critical and imminently lethal one. The reported profound prolonged QT and QTc values can be a precursor to ventricular tachycardia as well as torsades de pointe and can result in sudden cardiac death. This cardiac tracing associated with severe hypokalemia, hypoglycemia, hypomagnesemia and metabolic alkylosis should bring terror to treating clinicians.

Maryanna began her eating disorder while attending a private school. She boarded at the school in her hometown as her parents were living overseas on a military base near war zones. Safety was an issue.

At school she wanted to join the rowing team. The rowing team was made up of two weight categories. She weighed between these two categories. She chose to compete for the lower weight one. To do this she restricted faithfully. She did lose weight but began to binge eat in response to restricting. This, of course, led to vomiting to compensate for the excess food she was consuming and to, hopefully, further lose weight. Vomiting became a convenient way to eat whatever and how much she wanted and yet continue to lose weight. These behaviors stuck for over two decades.

Contributing to the body image control drive was that she became a model, a career that requires exacting body shape and weight control. Added to this is that she became an exotic dancer, a career that puts a focus on beauty as well as lean body shape. Modeling and exotic dancing brings with them sexualisation of body image.

Discussion

Maryanna's story is an unusual one. I spent many late night waking hours worried whether I was doing the right thing or not regarding my decision to monitor her the way I had.

A significant issue in her management was that I was on thin ground threatening to have her picked up by the police or paramedics if she did not got go to the ER due to critical lab values. It behoves us to contact our licencing bodies to determine our legal rights and obligations. In the end, it becomes an ethical or "the right thing to do" decision regardless of the laws of the land. Ethical decisions and legal statutes do not necessarily align.

Remarkably, after a couple of decades of Maryanna harbouring a severe eating disorder where there had been countless times she should have died, she fully recovered and attained a healthy weight for her age. She married and invited me to her wedding.

Lesson Points

- The tipping point for lethal outcomes, with regard to symptoms, critical medical laboratory values or cardiac status, is very individual. We cannot trust symptoms or medical investigations to accurately indicate risk. One individual's medical safety zone can be another's lethal one.

• Laws regarding certification or the capacity for clinicians to have individuals treated against their will, are determined by national and regional laws as well as local standards of care.

• The ethical need to treat may fly in the face of laws of the land.

• Maryanna's story is one that should have ended in disaster. Her medical status was unrelentingly critical almost daily for several years. Many others in similar situations could have died for sure.

• Control of body image with requisite weight and body shape expectations can be associated with ones sexual worth as defined by themselves and others. Some will enter the sex trade as a result, complicating their lives even more.

Elizabeth's Story

While in my office, I received a call from a father who said his daughter had been admitted to the ICU. The daughter had an eating disorder and was being treated for severe hypokalemia. The father stated that his daughter had a potassium level of 1.4 mmol/L. I wanted to say to him that he must have gotten the potassium value incorrect from the doctor as I was certain this was a blood concentration level that could not sustain life, however, I kept my thoughts to myself. I suspected he meant 2.4 mmol/L instead. I had never heard of a potassium level so critically low even after a couple of decades of experiences with those with eating disorders. Sure enough, his statement was accurate. I sent for a copy of the hospital lab reports and confirmed his assertion.

Elizabeth was a 28 year-old young woman, 5 feet 11 inches tall, 95 lbs with a BMI of 13.2. She worked as a librarian at the university. Her eating disorder behaviors included severe nutrition restriction as well as frequent binging and vomiting other times. Complicating her medical status was that she developed a pulmonary embolism. She required INR readings (International Normalized Ratio or prothrombin time) taken regularly to assure the dosage of her anticoagulant medication was in a therapeutic range. Unfortunately, she would not reliably comply with taking medications, having blood monitoring done, and it became impossible to contact her at times when critical lab values were reported for electrolyte or INR readings. Her cell phone would often be dead or she would just not respond to voice messages relaying life-threatening lab values. Family and friends were contacted who could have relayed messages to her, but were themselves often unable to locate her as she lived in her car at some undisclosed location. This was a nightmare scenario for myself and her family doctor who had been trying to reach out and manage her potentially lethal medical status. It was only with some luck that she would, indeed, contact us and comply with recommended treatments.

Discussion

A lesson I learned from my experience with Elizabeth and her father was to never assume I knew the extremes of medical compromise created by an eating disorder for any one individual. Also, this experience reaffirmed my mantra to *expect the unexpected*. The development of a pulmonary embolism, a condition not related to the eating disorder, further complicated her medial risks. On top of this, her unreliability with regard to monitoring and the inability of caregivers being able to contact her with critical laboratory values upped the potential risks even further. Clinical situations seldom become scarier than this.

When medical risks become seemingly impossible to resolve, they may do so on their own without our help. Although Elizabeth became lost to our follow-up, she ended up coming under the care of a family that nurtured her, providing employment, and shelter. It is also likely she was having her medical care managed elsewhere by this time. Sometimes, in medicine, if it weren't for dumb luck, we wouldn't have any luck at all.

I remember a quote from the musical *Fiddler on the Roof* where the grandson is riding with his grandfather in a horse drawn carriage. The grandson says to the grandfather "Grandfather, do you believe in miracles?" The grandfather says "No. But I depend on them." In healthcare, sometimes we do, indeed, have to depend on miracles from time to time.

Lesson Points

- *Never assume* to know the extremes of medical compromise from eating disorder and non-eating disorder health issues.
- Expect the unexpected. Never think, "It can't get any worse."
- If previous attempts to contact patients or significant others haven't worked, keep trying. Have significant others keep trying as well and get them to inform you if they have been successful.
- Dumb luck is our friend sometimes.

Maya's Story

This is the story of Maya, a 17 year-old young woman in grade 11, who likely died of complications of an eating disorder. Below are comments made by the coroner.

"She lived at home with her parents and two sisters. She was downstairs watching TV when one sister came down to join her and found her sitting, leaning on her hand apparently watching TV. Maya was totally unresponsive. Resuscitation was attempted by paramedics but she was pronounced dead in the ER. Maya dieted on and off since she was 15 years old.

The post mortem revealed extensive bilateral subconjunctival hemorrhages.

The respiratory tract revealed a mass of undigested food impacted in the lower trachea and both bronchi. The appearance in the lungs were consistent with ensuing asphyxia. Small petechiae were present over the pericardial surface characteristic of asphyxia. The esophagus showed congestion in the lower one-third. The stomach contained a mass of undigested and partially digested food which when removed it was noted extensive mucosal congestion with areas of interstitial hemorrhage present. In some areas there appeared to be superficial splitting of the gastric mucosa notably in the middle one-third of the stomach suggestive of violent gastric spasms and contractions. This would be consistent with vomiting.

The microscopic sections of the gastric mucosa confirmed the presence of vascular congestion with areas of extravasation of blood into the covering mucosa. Sections of the lungs revealed extensive severe congestion. The debris found in the lungs was consistent with aspiration of gastric contents.

The investigation revealed that she died as a result of aspiration of food contents. Evidence on autopsy related to violent vomiting having occurred. However, there was no vomit noted at the scene when she was found. Her family did not hear any choking sounds or noise of any kind from her. When she was found, her position was normal and relaxed as if she was quietly watching television. The paramedics did not visualize any obstruction in the upper airway prior to intubation but felt her lungs were tight.

It is unusual for a conscious neurologically competent individual to die from asphyxia due to aspiration of gastric contents. It is possible she experienced nausea and vagal inhibition of the heart immediately prior to vomiting causing her to faint while seated in the chair. She may then have aspirated as her airway was unprotected while unconscious."

Just prior to her death, she was having a competition with her sister to see who could lose the most weight before going on a holiday to Italy in a few weeks.

Discussion

Maya's story is an unusual one to say the least. Here is another example of a young person who had been diagnosed with an eating disorder after death. There were no previously known indications of an eating disorder noted by her family or family doctor.

What was not screened for was evidence of emetine, the active ingredient in Ipecac. Ipecac could have been responsible for creating a lethal cardiac dysrhythmia that lead to her death. She could have also had a pre-existing cardiac electrical abnormality making her more susceptible to a cardiac event triggered by electrolyte and mineral compromise or Ipecac ingestion. There had been no indication of drug or alcohol usage.

What is suspected from the coroner's report is that Maya had been dieting and possibly began vomiting to cause weight loss before going to Italy. Additional eating disorder behaviors such as the use of laxatives, diuretics or both could have aggravated metabolic instability. Other contributing factors may have been the use of appetite suppressants or metabolism boosters, both of which could have had an excitatory effect on the heart contributing to the risk of sudden cardiac death.

Lesson Points

- Clinicians need to be aware of all of the medications or ingested chemicals that can have an effect on cardiac function.
- Too many individuals die of complications of an eating disorder before others are aware the eating disorder existed.

Brenda's Story

I never met Brenda but I had chatted with her sister by phone regarding severe anorexia nervosa. She and her sister lived in a small town too far away for Brenda to come to our eating disorder program for treatment. She refused to accept medical help in her hometown. Brenda declined attending the tertiary eating disorder program in a bigger center as well. Following is what the coroner reported regarding her death.

"This 43 year old woman had a long history of severe anorexia nervosa. In the 2 to 3 months preceding her death, her weight took a significant drop. She was depressed for the last few weeks and refused medication and medical intervention. She collapsed and was pronounced death shortly after being taken to the hospital.

She weighed 39 kilogram (86 lbs) The body was extremely emaciated and there was virtually no subcutaneous fat and almost no soft tissue on the limbs. The abdomen was protuberant. There was a small amount of abnormal hair growth on the face.

On internal examination there was approximately one litre of straw coloured fluid in both pleural cavities and approximately three litres in the abdominal cavity. The uterus and ovaries were atrophic. There was a large stag-horn calculus in the left renal pelvis that obstructed the proximal ureter. There were numerous calculi in the right ureter. There was marked hydronephrosis and the cortex of each kidney was very thin and pale.

Microscopic examination of the heart showed focal degenerative change in the myocardial cells. Sections of the kidneys show atrophy of the cortex, scarring and patchy chronic inflammatory infiltrate in the interstitium. The section of the ovary showed mild ovarian atrophy.

Changes in the heart and ovary are consistent with severe malnutrition. The changes in the kidneys are the result of the ureters being obstructed by stones. These stones were the result of the metabolic disturbances produced by the severe malnutrition this woman suffered."

Discussion

Brenda's story is one of many in society who refuse treatment for their eating disorder and resulting medical decline. A question arises as to whether she should have been certified as mentally incompetent? Legally, could she have been certified as it would be clear to a judge that she knew exactly the risk factors from her behaviors including death? This is akin to an alcoholic who develops potentially lethal consequences of excessive alcohol drinking. Authorities never certify an alcoholic regardless of the lethality of their alcohol excess behaviors. Therefore, it has been pretty much the same for those with eating disorders. It is important for clinicians to be aware of laws regarding certification of those with eating disorders. There are laws that have been made in recent years, in some legal jurisdictions, that state those with life-threatening eating disorders must be certified or treated against their will in order to save their lives. Physicians should consult with their medical protective association's legal department.

Lesson Points

- Consider certification for those with severe and life-threatening health risks from an eating disorder. You may or may not be successful with this process.
- Even if certified, there is a strong likelihood that they still may refuse treatment for medical compromise in the emergency ward. You won't know till you try it. Sometimes just keeping individuals alive in the short term is all we are left with.
- I have managed the care of individuals with severe, unrelenting medical decompensation who receive intermittent stabilization of metabolic, renal, and cardiac risks year after year who should have died a long time ago but instead end up improving a decade or so later. The message here is *never give up*.

Marissa's Story

Marissa, a fifteen-year old girl, first came to see me in my office with a nasogastric tube coming out of her nose. She was accompanied by her mother, a single parent. They had driven over two hours from another town for the appointment.

Marissa was being tube fed nasally by her mother because every time she ate she developed left lower quadrant pain. She was fed a homemade liquid nutrition concoction at night while she was sleeping.

Marissa had been hospitalized six times in her hometown as well as twice at a tertiary care pediatric eating disorder program in a major center. Marissa would be hospitalized because of precipitous weight loss and then be renourished. Admission to the tertiary care center was arranged in order to provide concentrated expert eating disorder management. She was referred to me by her family doctor for an assessment of her medical status as well as eating disorder. I admitted Marissa to a general pediatric ward twice over a few months.

During each visit I consulted a pediatrician, dietitian, and gastro-enterologist. The pediatrician was involved to manage any serious health risks and the gastroenterologist was consulted to assess and manage her abdominal pain. She eventually would accept nourishment delivered by nasogastric tube as well as normal eating in the hospital.

During the last few days of her second admission I said to Marissa, "In order to get over the eating disorder, you are going to have to deal with body image dissatisfaction triggers. That is, to not feel the need to control your weight." She said she had never been dissatisfied by her weight. Not ever. Her mother was present and confirmed her assertions. It was then that I experienced this sinking feeling in my chest that she did not have an eating disorder. She had never been on a weight loss diet. Her mother said that she never talked about her weight or about wanting to go on diets. I then said to the two of them, "Marissa, you do not nor have you ever had an eating disorder." The mother threw up her hands and said "That's what we've been trying to tell the doctors all this time." I think most patients and parents would have been angry with me for initially misdiagnosing their daughter but Marissa and her mother were actually most grateful for me figuring it out in the end.

What do you call a medical consultant? Someone to share the blame with at the last minute. I quickly consulted a general surgeon and gynecologist to screen her for causes of abdominal and pelvic pains. There was no definitive diagnosis found after all investigations, which was a relief at some level knowing nothing serious had been missed. We were still stuck with what was causing this pain, however. In retrospect, it might have been advisable to have a laparoscopic visualization of her lower abdomen and pelvis particularly to rule out endometriosis. Inflammatory bowel disease, diverticulitis, Hirschsprung's disease, bowel infections, hernias, and other potential causes of gut related pain had already been ruled out.

Discussion

How was it possible Marissa experienced ten hospital admissions having an incorrect diagnosis of anorexia nervosa? There are a number of possibilities for which this could have happened.

An Anorexia Nervosa Persona

Marissa came to our program and demonstrated several expected personality manifestations of someone with anorexia nervosa. Although not all those with eating disorders present with one set of typical personality traits, there are characteristics common to many. It's human to make assumptions regarding individuals based on preset expectations.

Marissa presented cooperative and quite non-verbal. She let her mother speak for her seemingly not disagreeing with her mother's description of the reasons that led them to this visit. Those with anorexia nervosa can be rather passive up front and quite endearing. They tend to say nothing rather than argue to the contrary. Needless to say, there are certainly exceptions to this one-dimensional descriptor. Marissa fit my conscious and likely subconscious picture of someone with anorexia nervosa. I had made a preemptive diagnosis within the first few minutes without having heard much history. I suspect that the other physicians who had been involved with her care such as her family physician, pediatricians, and emergency physicians had done the same. "Looks like a duck, swims like a duck..."

We Believe the "Experts"

Who isn't going to trust the conclusions of the "experts" from designated eating disorder programs including and especially those from tertiary care programs? My own fault here was trusting the admitting and discharge histories reported from Marissa's admissions to a tertiary care specialized pediatric hospital program. I would have read these consult notes but did not scrutinize them for accuracy regarding diagnostic criteria. It was clear after rereading these notes that the attending pediatrician must have assumed she had anorexia nervosa from her anorexic persona, restricting behaviors, significant weight loss as well as related signs and symptoms and not because of a meticulous history that could have easily ruled out a diagnosis of anorexia nervosa. Nowhere in the consult notes had there been a clear and definitive assessment mentioned regarding body image dissatisfaction, a strong desire to lose weight, or weight control behaviors prior to hospitalizations.

Absence of Detailed Body Image Dissatisfaction, Weight Control Drive, or Diet History

All hospital consult notes, including my own, had failed to include an exquisite body image dissatisfaction, weight control drive, or diet history. All of us must have passed over this part of the assessment unaware having already decided she had an eating disorder.

Abdominal and Pelvic Pain Was Atypical

Almost everyone with anorexia nervosa has some form of abdominal pain from time to time. Abdominal pain often comes with having eaten something especially after prolonged restricting. It could be caused by the type of foods eaten. Some experience abdominal pain with eating protein, spices, fats, or other nutrients. Intestinal dysmotility is a primary cause of abdominal pain in those with eating disorders. The discomfort is usually epigastric and upper abdominal generally. Left lower quadrant pain is atypical.

Marissa's Case Was Not Reevaluated After Each Admission

Every time someone with an eating disorder is to be readmitted for eating disorder or medical assessment, a total unbiased evaluation should take place. Possibly for every readmission that Marissa undertook, there had been a "topped up" history where the admitting clinician would have tacked on the most recent concerns for readmission to previous poorly scrutinized assessment histories, discharge summaries, or treatment directives.

Enter Dr. Bryan Lask!

Bryan Lask was, arguably, the most expert clinician in the field of pediatric anorexia nervosa for his day. He worked in London, UK, mainly at the Great Ormond Street Hospital's Eating Disorder Program. I helped to organize an international eating disorder conference for which Dr. Lask had been asked to be a presenter. We asked him to review our program and give input. He, in turn, asked us to present a case of someone with anorexia nervosa for all of us to discuss. I presented Marissa.

With Marissa and her mother present, Dr. Lask began to question Marissa about her suspected eating disorder. He had read her hospital summary notes. He asked a brief eating disorder related history then took a piece of paper and drew a single line on it. At the left of the line he put a zero and at the right of the line he put 100. He then asked Marissa to put an X on the line where she felt that she was dissatisfied with her weight. She put the X to the very left on the line. This indicated a near total lack of body image concern. Bryan then said to her, "You do not and have never had anorexia nervosa." This had been my conclusion. His assessment took literally under 10 minutes. I felt vindicated that I had made the right conclusion.

Ward Politics

Regardless of the fact that I had correctly excluded a diagnosis of anorexia nervosa, I experienced much grief from the attending pediatrician during

Marissa's last hospital admission. He did not agree with my or Dr. Lask's assertions.

So, What Did We Finally End Up Knowing About Marissa?

Marissa's mother was an RN. She worked for an international non-profit health organization. Prior to Marissa's eating and abdominal pain symptoms she and her mother had moved to southeast Asia to work with impoverished families. Sanitation was abysmal. Marissa, being a foreigner, was teased by the local children with rotting fish heads and other disgusting acts. Marissa started to restrict in Asia and carried on this behavior when returning home. She restricted not because of any body image concerns but because she was profoundly depressed. She also declined food because she had developed a true food aversion created by the teasing and horrible sanitation. Although a thorough abdominal and pelvic pain work-up had taken place, a proper diagnosis was never concluded due to lack of follow-up.

Lesson Points

- Before ascribing treatments for those with eating disorders, make an accurate diagnosis based on a very thorough assessment of diagnostic criteria. Especially nail down a hard body image dissatisfaction, weight control drive, diet and eating disorder behavior history. If there is not enough supporting history for anorexia nervosa, don't guess. Allow for *diagnosis to be determined* with an eating disorder tucked in the differential diagnosis.
- Consider the comments made by other clinicians in their consult notes as well as verbally but assess each person being evaluated for an eating disorder with a clean slate making sure a diagnosis is yours and yours alone.
- Be aware of the possibility of personal biases, including yours and others, leading to quick diagnoses.
- Pay attention to clients or parents that disagree with a diagnosis. There may be validity in their assertions as in Marissa's case.
- Don't be afraid to ask for the opinions of colleagues. They very well may support your impressions. They may also provide new and even contrary opinions that are helpful.
- A deliberate refusal to eat may have other causes than an eating disorder as in Marissa's situation.
- Abdominal pains, even if triggered by eating, may not be due to eating disorder etiology.

Donna's Story

Donna is a 24 year-old woman with a long history of abdominal and pelvic pains beginning when she was fourteen.

Her first symptoms began as vague but progressive pelvic pain that was intermittent at first then became chronic and persistent. Over time, she developed irregular periods and pain with intercourse. Her family doctor felt she might have endometriosis. Abdominal plain films, pelvic ultrasound, and CT scan were unremarkable. Urological causes for the pain were ruled out. A course of the oral contraceptive pill and then a hormonal intrauterine device did help the pain a bit but not much. She was referred to a gynecologist.

The gynecologist agreed that her pain was likely due to endometriosis. Donna's mother and older sister had endometriosis. Donna was booked for surgery and had a laparoscopy. No endometrial lesions were visualized. The pelvis looked very healthy. After it was suggested she remain on hormonal contraception the gynecologist referred Donna to a physiotherapy clinic where they could teach her how to do pelvic floor exercises. The pains, however, persisted.

Donna developed painful mouth and vaginal sores. At a clinic she was told she likely had a herpes simplex outbreak. Her partner accused her of being unfaithful. These sores resolved after a week. Swabs for herpes simplex virus and syphilis were negative. Coincidently she had been experiencing some intermittent diarrhea. She occasionally had some blood with a bowel movement. This was initially attributed to hemorrhoids that came and went. Abdominal pains were worse with eating which led her to restrict solids. She lost weight and, although hungry much of the time, continued to greatly limit nutrition intake. A short time after the oral and vaginal sores began, she noticed a significant increase in diarrhea, bloody stools, and abdominal pain. She also experienced night sweats. She was then suspected of having inflammatory bowel disease. A preliminary work-up revealed she was anemic and imaging showed significant indications of Crohn's disease. She was then referred to a gastroenterologist.

The gastroenterologist ordered further investigations. A sigmoidoscopy showed several ulcers in the colon suggesting ulcerative colitis but biopsy confirmed Crohn's disease. An upper GI series with follow-through demonstrated strictures in the small intestine. Endoscopy clearly showed ulcers in the esophagus, stomach and upper small intestine. Biopsies of the upper intestinal track confirmed a diagnosis of Crohn's disease.

Over the years, Donna had multiple surgical operations for complications of Crohn's disease. Twenty-six in total. Surgery was performed to remove sections of bowel due to strictures, chronic and unrelenting inflammation as well as inactive bowel. Fistulectomies were performed to remove perianal fistulas. Eventually her small and large bowel, stomach, and esophagus were removed. She was being nourished via a peripheral inserted central line or PICC line. It was after all this surgery that Donna was referred to me at the eating disorder program.

Donna could not stop herself from chewing and spitting food. She, of course, was not able to swallow food including liquids. She could not swallow her own saliva as well. Any food particles taken into the mouth would get trapped in diverticula in her throat that would, in turn, become infected leading to further hospitalizations. She was referred to me to determine whether she, indeed, had an eating disorder. Due to her work schedule we never met again after her initial assessment. I was unable to provide any support surrounding her concerns.

Discussion

Donna's initial abdominal and pelvic pain symptoms presented much like endometriosis, a logical assumption at that time. Crohn's disease was not investigated for until more overt gut symptoms developed such as diarrhea, bloody stools and symptoms of developing bowel obstruction. After multiple hospitalizations and surgical operations Donna was devastated with not being able to eat or even taste food. She engaged in chewing and spitting that she was unable to control. This led to throat diverticula becoming infected and forming abscesses.

Although chewing and spitting is a rather common eating disorder behavior for those with anorexia nervosa and bulimia, Donna did not have a true eating disorder. The reason for chewing and spitting was different. Her situation was, however, no less serious or important.

Lesson Points

- Donna was originally misdiagnosed with endometriosis. Because of this, she suffered for an extended period of time due to a lack of proper medical management.
- Chronic abdominal and pelvic pain needs to be investigated thoroughly in order to rule out non-eating disorder related etiology. These pains are often attributed to eating disorder behaviors and ignored until salient non-eating disorder signs and symptoms come to light. With regard to Donna, she was correctly not suspected of having an eating disorder.
- Though clinicians who focus on regular eating disorders such as anorexia nervosa and bulimia, will from time to time have individuals referred to them for other forms of disordered eating. It can be our task to address these as well. There may be, however, strict guidelines that eating disorder programs and individual clinicians adhere to being expected to treat only those with true eating disorders.
- Those who develop aberrant eating behaviors, triggered by non-eating

disorder health concerns, may adopt body image control attitudes and behaviors subsequently. As an example, someone who acquires a severe gastroenteritis after touring a foreign country, may receive accolades for losing weight and compliments on how good they look as a result of weight loss caused by vomiting, diarrhea, and nausea resulting in food avoidance. They may then wish to further lose weight and deliberately restrict, over-exercise or vomit to continue a trend of losing weight. Any health issue that affects eating or weight may lead to full-on eating disorder attitudes and behaviors.

- Any complaints regarding abdominal pain and other seemingly gastro-intestinal symptoms such as nausea, vomiting, and diarrhea need to also be investigated for reproductive organ origins. A *pregnancy test* is a must. There are few really catastrophic clinical decisions that can end in death and missing an ectopic pregnancy is one.
- For clinicians who work with those with eating disorders, expect that there could be two diagnostic etiologies for symptoms with every patient. One potential diagnosis is for symptoms originating from an eating disorder and another for a medical or psychological condition not related to the eating disorder. Certainly, an eating disorder can aggravate symptoms evolving from another origin such as pelvic pains secondary to Crohn's disease or depression preexisting the eating disorder. As well, non-eating disorder health issues can exacerbate symptoms of eating disorder origin. As an example, hyperemesis gravidarum could add to the vomiting frequency of someone with bulimia and endogenous depression could aggravate depressive symptoms resulting from disappointing body image and weight loss pursuits. Signs and symptoms certainly may be due to only one diagnosis but consider the possibility of others.

Gillian's Story

A three-year old girl refuses to eat. She pushes her plate of food away when presented to her.

Discussion

This story brings up several possibilities for a girl refusing to eat. One is that she has a medical condition that is inhibiting her desire to eat. Conditions such as cancer, the flu, an ear infection, and so forth are possible. There could be a psychological trigger such as depression or a history of trauma. Another scenario is that she is mimicking her mother's restricting eating disorder habits or she has a pediatric eating disorder. It may be that she is repulsed by food for any number of reasons including having been exposed to spoiled food or foods with bad odors. An absence of taste and smell that could diminish at-tractiveness to food may be due to head injury or a respiratory virus.

In this particular situation, the girl was mimicking her mother's restricting eating disorder behavior. She would see that her mother would not eat at meal times, so she did the same. To reverse this food refusal behavior, her mother needed to eat at meal times so her daughter would learn to model appropriate eating.

Lesson Points

- Children can adopt the eating patterns of others.
- Those who care for children and have an eating disorder need to keep their body image dissatisfaction attitudes to themselves and eating disorder behaviors out of sight of children. This goes for parents, siblings, aunts, uncles, grandparents as well as family friends and baby sitters. Even though a parent with an eating disorder will say "I'm only talking about myself when I say I should lose weight but never criticize my daughter's weight or eating habits," kids pick up other's body image dissatisfactions and can internalize these attitudes themselves.
- A three year old is likely to be copy-catting her mother's restricting behaviors and not reacting to her own body image concerns. However, having said this, very young children can develop body image dissatisfaction and express feeling fat leading them to groom body size and shape altering habits.
- If restrictive eating persists and is not due to body image or weight control issues in children, adolescents or adults, then an *avoidant/restrictive food intake disorder (ARFID)* diagnosis may need to be considered.

Leah's Story

This is the abbreviated story of Leah, a 19 year-old swimming instructor, as told in the corner's report.

"She was found unconscious and unresponsive by her parents on the floor of her ensuite of her bedroom. She was taken to the hospital by paramedics where she was pronounced dead. There was nothing obvious in her bedroom to suggest the mechanism of death. Several packages of laxative were, however, found. Largely because she perceived herself gaining weight, she had only eaten sparsely the last few days prior to her death.

A full autopsy revealed petechiae on the visceral pleura, a very non-specific finding and suggested terminal asphyxia. Detailed examination of the heart showed focal mild myocyte attenuation consistent with the history of dieting. Further investigation of the death scene showed large quantities of Ex-Lax in the bedroom. The vitreous potassium level was 8.1 and would be at the lower end of the reference range for this post mortem interval. Detailed analysis of the heart showed only focal mild myocyte attenuation. This would be consistent with dieting but since the changes were not widespread, it is difficult to believe that is was directly related to her death.

From the history and analysis of the death scene, it seems that she was suffering from an eating disorder, consistent with bulimia. It is highly likely that her death was related to electrolyte imbalance due to excessive laxative use. In support of this is the borderline low vitreous fluid potassium. Hypokalemia is a well-known complication of excessive laxative use. This in turn renders the heart more irritable and prone to fatal dysrhythmia."

Discussion

Leah likely had an eating disorder. What is tragic is that she was diagnosed with this after she died. Her family was unaware of the laxative abuse or other possible eating disorder behaviors.

The coroner was correct in assuming the low vitreous potassium could have been caused by laxative use. However, although there is no history or other evidence of this, she may have been vomiting as well contributing to potassium loss. We will never know. Potassium levels remain relatively preserved for some time in the vitreous fluid. Serum levels of potassium cannot be relied upon post mortem as red blood cells break down quickly after death and release potassium elevating serum potassium levels.

Lesson Points

•   There are an unknown number of those with eating disorders who just drop dead without anyone being aware that they have an eating disorder.
•   As clinicians, we need to have a high index of suspicion for those in our office or in the emergency room who demonstrate the slightest indication of eating disorder behaviors or possibly related medical symptoms and signs.

Esther's Story

Esther was a 24 year-old woman, when I first met her, who significantly restricted by not eating breakfast or lunch but did have something for dinner. She was vegan. She exercised over two hours daily, at a minimum, and often more as she was a triathlete. She occasionally used laxatives and vomited to prevent weight gain but not very often. She did not mention experiencing palpitation, shortness of breath, chest pains, or syncope. Her BMI was 16.5. Esther would run with her sister, who was also vegan, and a friend who were training as triathletes. Esther absolutely refused to decrease exercise or increase nutrition and flatly refused to want to recover.

She rarely allowed herself to be weighed. She did have a family physician who was monitoring her and obtained an EKG report showing a heart rate of

35 bpm. The QTc was 500 msec. The EKGs were otherwise normal. I felt that her heart rate was unusual as it was always being recorded at 35 bpm with no variability. There would normally be some variation of heart rate expected whether the bradycardia was caused by the eating disorder, athletic endeavors, genetics or, very possibly, a combination of these. Could there be yet another etiology? Electrolyte, mineral levels as well as all other blood and urine screening was normal. I requested a thorough cardiac assessment through her family doctor.

A repeat EKG showed isorhythmic dissociation and competing junctional rhythm – a finding not observed previously. She was then referred to a cardiologist. A 24 hour holter monitor showed frequent ectopic atrial beats and occasional junctional escape beats. There were also rare ventricular ectopic beats and isolated PVCs. Her longest PR interval was 2.1 seconds. A transthoracic echocardiogram showed a secundum atrial septal defect with left to right ventricular shunting of uncertain QP/QS ratio. The atrial septal defect was at least 8.0 mm with right ventricular dilation. The cardiologist stated these finding were "concerning." A very mild mitral valve prolapse (MVP) had also been diagnosed that had not been noticed prior. A transesophageal ultrasound was recommended but it is not known whether this procedure had been carried out or not due to lack of follow-up. A percutaneous closure device was recommended. The cardiologist suggested she limit her exercise, increase her nutrition and avoid laxatives and vomiting.

Discussion

Esther represents yet another individual who declines to accept that her restrictive eating, laxative use, occasional vomiting, and exercise regime were risks to her health. What was unusual about Esther's bradycardia is that there was little if any variation in the 35 bpm rate. Further investigation proved fruitful with the discovery of an atrial septal defect and MVP.

Regardless of the individual's lack of acceptance of having an eating disorder or refusal to accept management of it, persistence by clinicians proved useful. Although Esther would not accept attention to eating disorder health risks, she did allow investigations of cardiac concerns.

The initial drive for competitive athletic endeavors likely had nothing to do with the eating disorder originally. However, exercise did evolve as a weight control device later. Laxative use was stated to be for occasional relief of constipation and that may be its whole intended purpose. However, laxative use could also have become a convenient way to lose weight. With further questioning regarding vomiting, Esther says she vomited infrequently only to control overwhelming negative feelings she experienced as a result of sexual assault.

The finding of a mild MVP opens the door to the possibility of potentially serious and life threatening health risks. The MVP may have associated with it occult aberrant electrical pathways that may create serious and even lethal dysrhythmias. The finding of an isorhythmic dissociation and competing junctional rhythm that seemed to have come from nowhere, and had never been observed before, sparks a need for close cardiac monitoring. This finding could be an early warning sign or beacon of more serious cardiac pathology yet to come to light.

Lesson Points

- Persist with medical monitoring and further investigations with the resistant client when possible.
- It may be necessary to have all discussion regarding nutrition, weight or eating disorder behaviors off the table for a while in order to be allowed to focus on pure medical concerns.
- Any evidence of a mitral valve prolapse, no matter how minimal, must be followed closely from the beginning and considered a potentially lethal threat as a result of associated dysrhythmias. Minor MVP etiology can become worse on it's own and also because of progressing medical compromise as a result of eating disorder actions.

Sharon's Story

Sharon was a 28 year-old woman who would often collapse to the floor a few times a month. Being a laboratory technician for a biotech company, she worked in an environment where there were concrete floors and stainless steel counters. She had just recently been accepted to medical school and would, therefore, become responsible for the care of others, a career where she could not ever sporadically collapse unconscious. By the time I first met Sharon, she had lost over 55 lbs within the previous year with a 30 lb weight loss just in the last 3 months. She dropped weight from 162 lbs to 101 lbs. She was 5'7". Her BMI reduced from 25.4 to 15.8. She was diagnosed with anorexia nervosa. Her only eating disorder behaviors were restricting and compulsive exercising. Syncope with loss of consciousness had occurred for years prior to losing weight.

Sharon was assessed by a cardiologist. She wore an event monitor for two weeks and it documented runs of supraventricular tachycardia (SVT) and rare atrial ectopic beats. There were no experiences of palpitations or loss of consciousness during these episodes. They occurred when she was sitting. An echocardiogram revealed a mild mitral valve prolapse. There had been no auscultation indication for the MVP. All other investigations were normal. The cardiologist concluded that she was experiencing vasovagal events and that she had a benign cardiac condition. She was allowed to work and drive regardless of syncope. The cardiologist recommended she increase fluids to improve hydration and consume more salt. This regime seemed to have been successful in conjunction with improved nutrition as well as adequate weight gain. The mild mitral value prolapse remained.

Discussion

It is not surprising that an individual who has lost so much weight and was likely quite dehydrated would have syncopal events. However, syncope and loss of consciousness occurred long before she experienced weight loss and before the eating disorder began. The runs of SVT recorded by the event monitor were not associated with symptoms. It calls into questions what cardiac patterns may or may not be occurring during periods of syncope and lose of consciousness.

I am not sure that her condition has been truly proven to be benign. I worry that she may have an undiagnosed source for the dysrhythmias and that it could have lethal potential as she became older. Could there be a genetic or acquired cardiac anomaly affecting the electrical conductivity of her heart? Is the mitral valve prolapse also associated with an aberrant electrical network? Could this be a similar scenario discussed for Erica where coronary athero-sclerosis and myxoid deposition were only identified at autopsy? Because Sharon had moved on and recovered from the eating disorder, I did not have any further contact with her. I would, however, have wanted her to have repeated Holter or event monitoring if symptoms remained or progressed.

Lesson Points

- Any cardiac or other cardiovascular findings (dysrhythmias, syncope, shortness of breath or chest pain) that disappear on their own or with medical support (renourishment or medications) should still be monitored closely. Repeat cardiac investigations should take place from time to time regardless of a lack of symptoms. The reason being that there could be an occult underlying pathology that had been aggravated by weight loss and nutrition compromise that still remains, posing a possible threat in the future.
- Mitral valve prolapse is sometimes associated with aberrant electrical conductivity induced dysrhythmias that may progress to lethal outcomes. They may be genetic or acquired. Mitral valve prolapse may exist before an eating disorder begins and may progress due to weight loss thus compromising the heart further. Mitral valve prolapse may develop for the first time as a result of significant weight loss when the heart muscle mass will shrink. This alters the physical and functional dynamics of the mitral valve unit. Weight restoration usually reverses this process.

Rosemary's Story

Rosemary is a 21 year-old woman with a history of severe food restricting and vomiting. She did not engage in binge eating or use any other eating disorder behaviors. She had been diagnosed with anorexia nervosa.

With seeing her for the first time, I took a screening eating disorder history. When enquiring regarding possible eating disorder behaviors she had been utilizing, she revealed that she severely restricted food intake. I asked her when the last time she had eaten or drunk anything. She replied with "Two days ago." With further questioning, she said that she had been vomiting over this same two-day period. She used Ipecac, a commercial emetic, to induce vomiting as she was unable to trigger vomiting without it. I asked her how much and how frequently she used Ipecac syrup. She said she used 6 bottles a day faithfully including over the last few days.

There is obviously a disconnect in her history in that why was she inducing vomiting when she had not been eating or drinking? I asked her "What are you trying to vomit?" She said "Air." She was inducing vomiting to rid her stomach of air in order to decrease the girth of her abdomen that, in her mind, made her look fat. She was able to remove air temporarily from her stomach six times a day this way.

Discussion

Rosemary's story demonstrates the extremes individuals will go to in order to control a perceived "fat" body image. Anyone looking at her would only see an emaciated figure and wonder how she could possibly see herself as over-weight. Her sense of having a fat abdomen may have been, in part, the result of the physical feeling of bloatedness and resulting distended abdomen. Abdominal pain or cramping may have contributed to her fears of being obese.

Ipecac was a commercially manufactured emetic that could be initially purchased over the counter in pharmacies then later behind the counter but always without the need for a prescription. It has since been taken off the legitimate drug store market and is not available in pharmacies. It is still available in use with alternative medicine practices.

Ipecac is a dangerous compound. The active ingredient in it is emetine. It is a myotoxin. Even with very small quantities but taken on a regular basis, it accumulates in muscle tissue over time, including the heart, similar to heavy metals such as lead can. This can lead to cardiomyopathy and electrical conductivity damage resulting in dangerous and lethal dysrhythmias. Ipecac has been reported to be fatal in as little as two bottles a week. Rosemary had been taking six bottles a day! Rosemary was found unconscious on the street one day. She was taken to the hospital to recover in intensive care. It was suspected that she may have become unconscious due to a serious dysrhythmia possibly triggered by emetine. When she woke up in the hospital, she had complete memory loss. She could not remember her mother, myself, or any events that should have been familiar to her. Coincidently, she had forgotten her eating disorder. She ate whole-heartedly and did not make any attempts to restrict or vomit. As her memory returned, so did her eating disorder attitudes regarding body mage self-loathing as well as restricting and vomiting behaviors.

Aside from toxicity, emetics can cause extreme forcefulness of vomiting to the degree that it results in renting of the stomach or esophagus. This could lead to exsanguination.

Lesson Points

• Never underestimate the extremes those with eating disorders will go to in order to fulfill their body image desires.
• Although Ipecac has been taken off of the market, other effective emetics are easily at hand. High concentrations of salt dissolved in water or eating mustard can be effective with regard to inducing vomiting.

Janet's Story

Janet is a 31 year-old woman five months pregnant. She was referred to me by her psychiatrist due to a significant lack of expected weight gain and fears that this was going to put her baby at risk of failure to thrive or premature labor. She was not gaining weight due to restricting. The reason for restricting was not clear. She did not relay any overt body image control concerns but fear of weight gain was considered in the differential diagnosis. She did not have any body image or weight control concerns prior to becoming pregnant.

I acquired a general eating disorder history as well as a medical history. I asked her regarding any experiences of sexual abuse or other regretted sexual experiences as I do 100% of all those referred to me. She went on to tell me about repeated sexual assault years earlier. This topic became the focus of our sessions subsequently. With addressing her assault concerns, she seemed to improve in mood and began to eat a bit better. One day she said to me "You're making me sick" with regard to continuing the focus on the assault issues. I said "Got it!" and never returned to this topic again. I did say that if she ever wanted to discuss it further, I would be open to this. We discussed local resources for those with a history of sexual assault.

One day she said she wanted to go home and that her mother would take care of her including providing meal support. She was tired of being on the maternity ward. She promised she would gain weight at home. With careful consideration, and consultation with the obstetrician, perinatologist, and psychiatrist I agreed to discharge her home for a one week trial. As she and her baby were currently stable and not at immediate risk, this seemed reasonable. If she, however, did not improve her nutrition with appropriate weight gain she would have to be readmitted.

I never saw Janet again for clinical follow-up. I assumed she was doing OK. I incidentally saw her on the mother-babe ward months later as I had just attended a deliver for one of my maternity patients. I did a lot of prenatal, delivery, and post-delivery management in those days. Her baby was delivered term and healthy. Janet looked well nourished and healthy.

Discussion

Pregnant woman can have eating disorders too. The eating disorder will typically have predated the pregnancy. In Janet's situation her disordered eating was never knowingly associated with body image control drives. I made the conclusion that her restricting behaviors were directly related to emotions stemming from the sexual assaults. These emotions and probably memories erupted after conception for unknown reasons. Regardless, addressing the abuses helped to relieve guilt, shame, and feelings of being responsible for what happened.

I have dealt with sexual abuse and other regretted sexual experiences for over three decades. I'm quite comfortable bringing up the topic and clients usually seem open to engaging in discussion. There are those, of course, who do not wish to go in this direction and may decide to discuss this with another clinician.

When bringing up the topic of sexual abuse I will say "Tell me what you are comfortable with or at least willing to talk about regarding this issue. If you don't want to talk about it, fine. I'll leave it up to you whether to discuss it at a later date or not." I have never enquired as to "What happened?" It is surprising how up front individuals are willing to chat if they are provided a safe environment to do so. In Janet's situation I had persisted a bit too much where my bringing up the subject was making her ill. Asking about abuse issues is the right thing to do. No one in the last thirty years was ever devastated by my enquiring nor have I ever regretted making enquires regarding sexual assault. If the clinician has a good connection with the individual, he or she will let you know if they have had enough discourse.

Lesson Points

- Pregnant women can have any version of an eating disorder.
- Disordered eating, whether body image focused or not, can begin during pregnancy for the first time.
- Never be afraid to bring up the subject of sexual assault or other regretted sexual experiences. Thoughtful and respectful discussion is the currency to having individuals open up.
- Unless a clinician has expertise in this area, refer to other clinicians or support groups that do.
- When enquiring regarding sexual issues we need to ask about sexual

assault as well as other regretted sexual experiences. Not all regretted sexual experiences are without consent. Individuals may engage in sexual activities perfectly willingly without coerced consent or while inebriated. Some will have desired sexual experiences and then regret it later. A fully consensual sexual act can be regretted and bring similar shame as nonconsensual sex. We need to ask regarding this.

- For many pregnant women, dealing with the eating disorder becomes naturally a bit easier. The reasons for this are not known. There is certainly a need to be "good for the baby" during pregnancy. There is sometimes a kind of reprieve. Concern comes, however, after delivery when the green light to engage in all-out eating disorder behaviors becomes possible. This is to make up for weight gained during pregnancy and pressures to have to be good for the baby for so many months. The postnatal period is a time for clinicians to be aware of potential impending eating disorder escalation.

Alita's Story

Alita was a 36 year old woman when I first met with her, presenting with intractable chronic pelvic pain. She had been diagnosed with anorexia nervosa as she wished to lose weight and, indeed, was emaciated when I first met her. She was referred to me by her gynecologist, requesting that I help her make a decision as to whether to perform surgery for endometriosis at this time. She was concerned whether Alita's medical status was stable enough for the procedure. Alita had been booked for a hysterectomy, bilateral oophorectomy and removal of all evidence of endometriosis within the pelvis assuming this would relieve her pain. There was a concern that Alita was addicted to morphine being used to control pain. Was there a chance she was faking pain in order to receive morphine? Being a mother of two children, it was imperative she become healthy enough to care for them. Alita's wife was able to manage things at home in the interim. Alita's screening health history revealed she had brittle insulin dependent diabetes mellitus (IDDM), hypothyroidism, and had a cholecystectomy after delivery of her first born.

Alita was unable to eat or drink anything due to food making her profoundly nauseated and often eliciting involuntary vomiting. This created a nightmare situation for managing the diabetes. On top of this, Alita developed a spontaneous pneumothorax that required a chest tube to be inserted.

This was becoming one of those medical "perfect storms." I was thinking "What next?" It was becoming clear something definitively had to be done very soon. This was an individual with severe emaciation, who could not eat or drink, with intractable pelvic pain who was dependent on morphine, *and* had a collapsed lung with resulting chest tube. Parenteral feeding had to be put in place. Management of her diabetes complicated things further. It became a critical decision point as to whether she was medically fit to undergo quite extensive surgery. The other option was to delay surgery until she had been renourished enough to decrease intraoperative and postoperative risk. The decision when to perform surgery was mine and mine alone. With much soul searching I concluded surgery should be done right away. Alita went through surgery successfully, began to eat and drink and was pain free aside from postsurgical pain. She did not require morphine for pain control and did not ask for it. Control of her diabetes became more manageable. She gained weight and became healthy as well as was able to care for her kids and return to work as a local television news anchor.

Discussion

Alita's story is a complicated and scary one. One compounding serious medical situation after another piled on, ramping up risk significantly each time. I remembered the wise words of a renowned intergalactic seer, "Do or do not. There is no try." These are the wise words of Yoda. There is a time when we have to put up or shut up. Or rephrased, pee or get off the pot. With all of the available facts in front of us and consultation with peers, we sometimes are left with a "best guess" scenario as to where to go next.

Out of all of Alita's medical risks, control of her diabetes became the worst risk factor. The urgency to get on with an immediate treatment solution was mostly based on the need to bring better control of the diabetes.

Lesson Points

- Chronic pain is a debilitating condition. It creates a sense of hopelessness and helplessness as well as breeds depression. It can have a negative effect on relationships including partners, children, and others. It can prevent someone from being able to go to work and may result in grave financial ruin. The medical bills accumulated in an attempt to control intractable pain with repeated failure to do so, can be staggering.
- Things can still get worse when already faced with near impossible medical situations. Never say "It can't get any worse than this." One of the themes of this book is *expect the unexpected*. This is no truer than faced with an already critical set of concerns.
- Even though emaciation, intractable pelvic pain, the lack of capacity to eat, and a collapsed lung were the upfront conditions that required attention, IDDM was the most dangerous complicating factor, a condition that predated all of the above.
- Sometimes individuals are dependent on pain medications not because

they are addicted to them but because they want pain relief. In effect, they are addicted to pain relief, not the medications that control it.

Danika's Story

Danika was a 24 year old woman who was admitted to a hospital based eating disorder program. She had been diagnosed with anorexia nervosa associated with unrelenting bingeing and vomiting behaviors. Aside from also being exercise compulsive, she was addicted to prescription diet pills. She would frequently doctor shop to receive a limited quantity of diet pills called Fastin or phentermine, an anorexiant used to cause weight loss and treat obesity. Many physicians were loath to prescribe this medication resulting in her having to visit several different doctors in a week.

One day she stole a prescription pad from the nursing station and wrote herself a prescription for Fastin to be filled at a nearby pharmacy. She did this as she had been denied the use of this medication on the ward. The pharmacist questioned the legitimacy of the prescription and reported this to the hospital where they said she had stolen the prescription pad and faked the signature. She was formally charged by police and had to appear in court.

After this event, I told her that diet pills do not work, at least for very long. Even in Fastin's own literature it is stated that it only works short-term to reduce weight. Weight would likely return. She said she didn't take Fastin to lose weight. She took it to make her sane. She described her mind as scattered and could not focus without this medication. Her story rang true. She may have had attention deficit/hyperactivity disorder (ADHD) and Fasten acted much like Ritalin and other related medications to control symptoms.

Discussion

This is a situation where the mantra, "Never assume. Always ask. Always know." applies. Certainly, individuals could use diet pills for both weight loss as well as mood stabilization.

Lesson Points

- Confirm with your patients their reasons for the use of each medication.
- Arrange for a psychiatric consultation with regard to undiagnosed psychological attitudes and behaviors possibly requiring medication management.

Carol's Story

Carol was 36 years old and worked as a pediatric anesthesiologist. She carefully restricted food intake and engaged in binging and vomiting daily. She did not dedicate any effort toward dealing with her eating disorder. She, however, had a longstanding addiction to alcohol. Her alcoholism had cost her much in her life. She was unable to keep a relationship due to being very undependable regarding keeping commitments and had multiple affairs she explained away as a result of being drunk. She had given birth to a baby boy but gave him up for adoption as she knew she could not care for him. She had also been charged with two DUIs. She lost her driver's license for one month and had to cab to work as well as elsewhere. She had become very skilled at hiding her drinking problem and the carnage she left behind because of it. She also had to leave a number of hospital jobs due to unreliability and had been threatened with losing her medical license if she did not clean up her act. Quitting one job and moving on to another in a different state helped her to dodge scrutiny by the medical college licensing body. Each hospital system gave her warnings regarding her alcoholism but never made efforts to bring formal disciplinary action. Every new anesthesia department that hired her was initially so grateful having her work for them that they never enquired as to her previous work track record. As far as was known, no harm had come to any patients.

One day Carol put a 11 year-old girl under anesthesia for surgery to remove her gall bladder. The girl became blue on the operating table and the surgeon questioned Carol if she had intubated the esophagus instead of the trachea. Carol was incensed by the assertion of the surgeon and insisted that the intubation had been done properly. Unfortunately, the surgeon had been correct. By the time Carol's error had been fully realized, the girl was brain dead.

Discussion

Carol had dodged the bullet of being discovered as a dangerous alcoholic so many times that the momentum of her potential lethality both with regard to driving intoxicated and working as an anesthesiologist went fully unchecked until it was too late.

She knew that her eating disorder and alcoholism coexisted together and, to her, were one and the same. She believed she did not need to seek help for either condition. Both served the same function which was to help her deal with life long anxiety as well as accumulating guilt and shame over hurt she had caused her friends, family and partners. Frequent moving due to changing employment caused her to become socially isolated as she had no friends or family to rely on in a new city. Her isolation and unbearable loneliness caused her to seek comfort further in her eating disorder, alcoholism and destructive relationships with other addicts.

Lesson Points

* For some, the eating disorder and chemical addiction feed off of each other and are used simultaneously to deal with the same life grinds.
* The medical crisis here was not experienced by Carol but created for the girl through Carol's own negligence.
* If the hospital administrations for each hospital had taken her incompetence seriously and acted decisively with regard to disciplinary action, the girl would not have died. The crisis would have been diverted.
* Those with eating disorders may have serious drug or alcohol addictions putting others lives at risk through their employment, driving a vehicle, or caring for children. Treatment for both the eating disorder and addiction should be insisted upon as soon as they have been identified.

Peggy's Story

Peggy, 27 years-old, was under my care for over two years for management of severe anorexia nervosa.

She restricted by eating less than 500 calories daily and walked for several hours every day. She would stick pins into various parts of her body that she felt were too fat with the superstitious thought this would release fat somehow. Her BMI was 12. She was emaciated and her skin was yellow likely from *carotenemia*. Though very medically compromised, she was able to work fulltime as an art therapist. She never, not once, followed any of my suggestions with regard to treatment but would attend appointments with me faithfully. She refused to be admitted to the hospital for medical monitoring, rehydration, or refeeding. She would not see a dietitian. She would also not have any laboratory testing. One day I told her that because she refused to engage in any of my recommendations that I would refuse to see her further. She would have to find another doctor for any medical issues. Two days later she ended up in the ER with profound rectal bleeding due to an opportunistic gastrointestinal infection and ended up in intensive care. Fortunately, the family physician on call, took her into her practice. Peggy later joined the newly funded eating disorder program locally and was followed by a therapist, psychiatrist, and dietitian. Although I was a clinician in this same program, I did not take on any part of her care. She did eventually agree to attend a tertiary care eating disorder program in another city. Regardless of this admission, she refused all treatment options offered as well and was discharged early. After over 25 years of care, she continued to refuse to engage in treatment. Her weight was just as low after over two decades as it had been when I first met her. Because of the lack of engagement in treatments offered, she was asked to take a time-out from the program but would be welcomed back if she decided to partake in treatment options. What is very surprising is that she lived as long as she did and remains alive into her late 50 s. All who cared for her over the years fully expected her to die of anorexia nervosa earlier in life but turned out to be wrong. Go figure.

Discussion

Of all the treatment offered by various clinicians in different cities, Peggy would not engage in any options offered for any length of time for almost three decades. She did, however, faithfully attend appointments for unknown reasons.

Lesson Points

- No matter how much care is offered there are some who will not ever engage in treatment even with clinicians' best efforts.
- There are some with severe medical compromise who clinically should have died long ago, but didn't.
- The body seems to be able to compensate for extremes of starvation defying what we know about nutrition and the functioning of the human body. For someone to claim to eat only 500 calories daily for decades as well as burn calories through over-exercising seems to defies scientific and medical logic.
- Regardless of Peggy's assertion she was only eating 500 calories daily, could she have been "cheating" on her severe restricting regime? Could she have been binge eating at times? Could her assessment of caloric intake been grossly inaccurate in the first place? A dietitian would have been able to sort this out.
- Regardless of the seemingly persistence of treatment refusal, it is possible that Peggy survived as long as she did because of decades long attention by caregivers.
- Refusing to offer care because of a client's reluctance to engage in treatment could be seen as unethical and possibly illegal by licensing bodies. It may be deemed abandonment. Be sure to check with your licensing body, colleagues, and treatment systems you may be employed with regarding declining care to clients.
- Regardless of how Peggy survived all these years with such seemingly high risks, we cannot become complacent with clients who are better nourished and possibly lower risk, as those with eating disorders may die at normal weights. Every individual with an eating disorder can have a very different threshold for demise when compared to others.

Fran's Story

I was contacted one day regarding a 71 year-old woman, Fran, who had been restricting and lost a lot of weight. The ward staff were concerned she had anorexia nervosa. I was very busy at the time and did not want to assess an elderly woman who, I felt at the time, could not possibly have developed an eating disorder in her 70s. I thought, however, that it would be likely faster to quickly see her and convince the staff she must have another medical issue causing restricted eating and weight loss such as depression, dementia or possibly a malignancy. Fran had just returned from attending a tertiary care center in another city having been referred there for assessment and management of severe osteoporosis. She had 6 collapsed vertebrae and was at risk of experiencing other fractures.

I met the woman and observed that she was emaciated. She was 5 feet 3 inches and 74 lbs. She had lost weight from 104 lbs a year earlier. The first thing I asked her was "Why are you not eating?" She said "Well, look at me. I'm so fat!" I think my jaw dropped to the floor. I could not believe what I had just heard.

With speaking to her family they said that Fran had never expressed any issue with her weight nor ever dieted prior to last year as far as they knew. Over this same time Fran had been becoming forgetful and would wander off from her home and become lost. It ends up that she was developing Alzheimer's disease. With development of the Alzheimer's symptoms, she coincidently developed a severely distorted "fat" body perception. There was no identifiable trigger to her disturbed body image.

Discussion

The idea of a woman, in her eighth decade, first developing a pathologically distorted body image with resulting deliberate food restricting behavior is remarkable. I would not have believed it if I had not witnessed it for myself.

The question is where did the "fat" awareness come from? Is it possible that with the development of Alzheimer's syndrome, a smoldering occult body image dissatisfaction was allowed to unmask itself? Was this a kind of disinhibiting process brought on by dementia?

Lesson Learned

- Never think you've seen or know it all.
- Body image dissatisfaction and resulting eating disorder can come to light for the first time in the geriatric population.

Annette's Story

Annette was referred to me because of body image concerns and some restricting eating behaviors. Her family doctor suspected she might have an eating disorder. She was just going into grade 11 but had difficulty engaging in classes and studying. A complicating factor that interfered with eating was significant head pain. She had had surgery for removal of a jaw cyst and at the same time had four molar teeth removed. She developed chronic facial pain ever since.

The facial pain affected Annette in a number of ways. Because the pain was chronic, she became depressed and unmotivated to participate in normal life expectations including those for school, practicing cello and spending time with friends. Her depression and general despondence amplified her self-loathing including hating her body. Pain also affected eating due to it increasing with chewing.

Discussion

Annette had two significant factors affecting eating. One was the combination of body image dissatisfaction, depression, and escalating self-loathing and, two, significant facial pain aggravated by chewing. She was referred to a pain clinic that seemed to be helpful. Attention to body-image dissatisfaction and restricting behaviors came later and were successful.

Lesson Points

*   A coexisting medical problem along side an eating disorder can, by itself, increase anxiety, depression, self-loathing, and a sense of hopelessness.
*   Attempts at working on eating disorder recovery are likely to be unsuccessful unless repressive medical issues are addressed in conjunction with eating disorder management or even before attending to eating disorder concerns.

Medication Complications and Eating Disorders

Medication complications can occur in those with eating disorders as with anyone else. Here are *Stories* that highlight medication concerns for some with eating disorders.

Lorrianne's Story

Lorrianne, an 18 year old woman, came to see me at a walk-in clinic because she had been told by her dentist that he would not work on her teeth unless she had seen a family doctor. The reasons for this were vague. Her medication review revealed she had been given a prescription for a narcotic to help her deal with dental pain. Almost all of her teeth had rotted to the gum line and extensive dental work under a general anesthetic was required. While in my office, she became unconscious and unresponsive. I gave her Narcan i.m. and she surprisingly very quickly came around and was alert. She informed me that she had taken the narcotic just before coming to my office and had never taken it before. The dosage was low and shouldn't have caused such a profound sedating effect.

The reason for her dentist refusing treatment became clear to me. Lorrianne was emaciated and possibly at increased risk of an anesthetic complication due to seriously compromised medical status.

I did a thorough physical examination and ordered blood and urine samples as well as an EKG stat. On examination she was very bradycardic, had frequent irregular heartbeats, and a systolic murmur. Her body was cachectic. Investigations revealed she was in metabolic alkylosis, was severely hypomagnesemic and anemic. An EKG displayed a heart rate of 32 bpm, a prolonged QTc interval of 580 msec and various irregular cardiac patterns including runs of PVCs and third degree heart block.

She was admitted to ICU and followed by an internist. A psychiatrist who specialized in eating disorders was consulted and when Lorrianne was medically stable, she was transferred to the psychiatric ward.

Discussion

Lorrianne had severe anorexia nervosa with profound restricting eating patterns as well as frequent binging and vomiting behaviors daily. She had become critically medically unstable by the time we had our first visit. Lorrianne's dental destruction was undoubtedly caused by frequent vomiting. The acid in her vomit would have caused her teeth to erode. She also had extensive gum damage. The cost of dental repair would be tens of thousands of dollars.

A contributing factor to the evolution of the eating disorder and a complicating factor to her recovery was that she had experienced horrific repeated sexual assaults.

Lesson Points

- Vomiting can cause extensive dental damage. Clinicians should examine the mouth of those with eating disorders thoroughly to look for any dental problems. Have your client consult a dentist regardless.
- Ask all those with eating disorders regarding possible sexual assaults.
- Lorrianne was exceptionally sensitive to the sedating effects of a narcotic. When prescribing any sedating medication and possibly other kinds of medications, ask regarding whether they have ever taken it before, and if they have, did they experience any reactions to it.
- Caution individuals regarding the additive and sometimes amplified affect of sedating medications when taken together. Discuss the risks of taking alcohol with sedating drugs including over the counter and illicit drugs.

- Those who have experienced major weight loss may be more sensitive to medications requiring much lower doses or none at all. Because metabolism may be altered significantly for those who are emaciated, various drugs from different classes may be metabolized differently depending on which enzyme pathways are required.
- The dentist refusing to treat Lorrianne unless a medical consultation had been carried out worked in her favor and may have saved her life.

Norma's Story

Norma, 17 years old, was dealing with severe anorexia nervosa. She restricted and over-exercised daily. She had a BMI of 14. She had been in and out of hospital both in her hometown as well at the tertiary care hospital in a major city. Admissions were primarily to deal with metabolic instability involving rehydrating and refeeding.

To deal with profound anxiety regarding having to improve nutrition both through nasogastric tube as well as orally, a potent anxiolytic was prescribed. She agreed to try this. The medication was a benzodiazepine, Valium or diazepam. Diazepam is a long acting benzodiazepine with a half-life of from 30 to 56 hours. It is particularly useful for chronic anxiety. Some other benzodiazepines have very short half-lives and may be used sparingly for dealing with acute anxiety in the moment. The shorter acting ones tend to be more addicting.

A dose of diazepam of 5–10 mg orally would likely cause significant drowsiness if not somnolescence in those not used to taking it. Norma was given 100 mg daily and this helped a bit to aid in nourishing. She, however, was very alert and showed no signs of affected gait, difficulty speaking or slowness of thought. When she returned to see me after discharge and I noticed the dose she was taking, I contacted her psychiatrist at the tertiary eating disorder program to confirm that this was the dose they had intended and, indeed, it was.

Discussion

Norma had an unusually high resistance to diazepam. This is the opposite reaction to what Lorrianne experience who was very sensitive to a low dose of a narcotic that put her into a coma.

Lesson Points

- Some with eating disorders may be very sensitive to normal doses of sedating medications and others may require exceptionally high doses to have any effect.
- It may be possible that a given individual may be hypersensitive to one medication and resistant to others.

- Regardless of the degree of sensitivity to any given sedating medication, caution against mixing it with other sedating medications or alcohol.

Sherry's Story

Sherry was a 32 year-old woman admitted to the psychiatry ward for management of an eating disorder. She had anorexia nervosa where she would restrict nutrition and over-exercise to control body image dissatisfaction as well as to deal with anxiety, depression, and memories of trauma. She was employed as a chiropractor but had to take time from work to attend hospital. Her fiancé was very supportive of her recovery.

With Sherry's best efforts and those of the treatment team, it became impossible to feed her either through oral or nasogastric means. She had intractable nausea. This created a serious issue because she was not even able to drink and keep fluids down. A nasogastric tube would not have remained in place due to vomiting. An I.V. line was installed so it would be possible to rehydrate her as well as supply minerals and electrolytes. It was decided that she would benefit from taking the anti-emetic, metaclopromide. It was delivered intravenously.

Soon after initiating metoclopramide, she was having hallucinations. She then developed painful muscle rigidity because of tardive dyskinesia. Metoclopramide was discontinued and she was given medication to reverse the symptoms of tardive dyskinesia.

Discussion

Sherry experienced serious side effects from metaclopromine. These side effects were important complicating factors when trying to restore nutrition and having psychological support for anxiety, depression and issues surrounding sexual abuse.

Lesson Points

- Would she have had these side effects regardless of having an eating disorder or had she become hypersensitive to this medication because of chronic starvation and significant weight loss?
- Side effects of medications can derail or at least delay existing treatment plans.

Stories of Suicide Attempts and One Suicide

Fiona's Story

I was asked to consult a 16 year-old young woman, Fiona, regarding her eating disorder. I brought her into my office from the waiting room and asked her why she was here. She said that she didn't think she had a problem with an eating disorder but came because her family pressured her to. Fiona confided right there in my office that she wanted to kill herself. I left my office momentarily to contact emergency mental health services in order to have her transported safely to the hospital for a psychiatric assessment. Upon returning to the office, Fiona was shoving a handful of pills into her mouth. She was so hurried to get as many pills into her mouth as possible that several were spilling to the floor. She was wanting to kill herself but I had caught her in the act of trying to suicide. Her overdose attempt had lethal intent. She was sent to the ER to be assessed by the psychiatrist on call. I never saw her again.

Discussion

Fiona had taken a handful or so of a selective serotonin reuptake inhibitor that her family doctor had prescribed for her. She did not realize that they were not particularly toxic and would not have died from her overdose attempt. If I had not returned to my office when I did, Fiona would have successfully taken as many pills as she intended without me being aware. If the medication had been toxic, she could have died sometime after leaving my office.

Lesson Points

- Clients can overdose anywhere, anytime.
- The reasons for her overdosing in my office rather than before or after our visit was never determined.
- Be sure to enquire regarding suicidal or self-harm ideation of every individual early on in assessment
- Be aware that no matter how much clinicians see themselves as trying to be helpful, our contact with clients can be triggering for reasons we may not be aware of.
- Our scheduled visits with clients could trigger suicidal acts before, during or after a given visit.

Pat's Story

Pat was an 18 year old you woman who came to visit me on my first day in my new practice. I had never seen her before. She had booked an appointment having been referred to me for concerns regarding a possible eating disorder. She seemed positive and upbeat. We had an introductory chat when I asked her why she had come to see me. She told me that she had taken a lethal dose of a sedative prior to coming. Trying to remain calm and supportive, I managed to get her to the ER for assessment by the emergency physician regarding medical complications of the overdose and psychiatric follow-up.

Discussion

Where Fiona had taken an overdose of pills *during* our visit, Pat had taken hers *prior* to coming to see me.

Lesson Points

- Both Fiona and Pat had taken overdoses in relation to their visits with me. The reasons for this are unclear. Were the overdose gestures a cry for help? Did their visit to me trigger a culmination of suicidal ideation? Did the overdoses have nothing to do with our appointments and were just coincidental? Did they not want to die alone?
- Look for signs of suicidal ideation in every client throughout the course of treatment.

Sonja's Story

Sonja was a 27 year-old woman with a long history of severe depression, anxiety, and anorexia nervosa. She was a survivor of child sexual abuse over many years. Her mother had been aware of the abuse but did nothing to stop it. She, in-fact, would slap Sharon on the face for not cooperating during rape sessions by the mother's partner. During her early teens, she became a permanent ward of Family and Child Services over a three-year period. After this, she became an emancipated youth, becoming legally independent from her parents and guardians. She had been seeing a psychologist for five years.

Coroner's Comments

"Sonja's medical history revealed basically good physical health. Her psychiatric history included a number of previous admissions to the psychiatric ward when she was a minor. Episodes of self-harm led to the admissions as well as a history of rapid weight loss and associated eating disorder. Documentation indicated Sharon was attempting to deal with a history of physical and sexual abuse.

Prior to her death, Sonja had been living with her boyfriend in a supportive stable relationship and she had many friends. She was attending university in her third year of anthropology.

She had a complete physical exam by her family doctor. At that time she complained of a small non-healing ulcer on her lower lip and weight loss of approximately 15 lbs in the past month. Her doctor felt she had an eating disorder and referred her to a nutritionist in the hospital. During their first visit, Sonja expressed concerns of acute suicidal thoughts. She had a history of overdosing with diuretics four times in the past. The dietitian walked her to the ER where she then became admitted to the psychiatric ward with a diagnosis of depression and suicidal ideation.

The ward psychiatrist's assessment confirmed a recent weight loss of 15 lbs with symptoms of depression, agitation, suicidal ideation, intense anxiety and anorexia nervosa. She experienced feelings of derealization and depersonalization. Approximately three to four weeks prior, she stopped eating due to body image becoming of great importance to her. Her weight had increased to 121 lbs and, therefore, panicked. Sonja felt her appropriate weight should be 118 lbs. She verbalized overwhelming fear of becoming fat to staff. Although her psychologist was not licensed to work in the hospital system she was allowed to see Sharon in the community utilizing three hour accompanied off-ward passes. She was encouraged to maintain nutrition on the ward.

Sonja's stay was tumultuous. She had several transfers from the main psychiatric ward to the Psychiatric Intensive Care Unit (PICU) because of acute suicidal intent. She told her psychiatrist that she wanted to hang herself in the women's washroom on the fourth floor. This was documented in the chart. Throughout her stay she repeated this desire. One day she brought a stereo speaker cord to the nurse's unit she had taken from the quiet room and was afraid she might use it to hang herself. She expressed to staff she was grateful the elevators were locked. She was started on fluoxetine with hopes of lifting depression to some degree.

One evening she went out on an accompanied pass with her boyfriend to have dinner. She bought a new dress and was proposed to. Earlier in the day, however, she had mentioned that she could not stand her weight. After returning to the ward, she was placed on a fifteen-minute suicide watch. She soon could not be found. A hospital wide alert was initiated as well as the city police were alerted. A patient came to the nursing station stating that someone needed help in the women's washroom adjacent to the common area. When the staff entered the washroom they found Sharon hanging by a white bathrobe belt from the bathroom stall. She was immediately cut down and found with no vital signs. Resuscitation attempts were unsuccessful.

The post mortem examination revealed "a ligature abrasion of the neck and pulmonary congestion. External examination revealed a weight of 56.4 kilogram (124 lbs) and height of 159 centimeters (5'3"). The immediate cause of Sonja's death was asphyxiation due to hanging. Contributing to her death were depression, suicidal ideation and eating disorder. Toxicology revealed a therapeutic level of chlorpromazine which was non-contributory to death."

Discussion

Sharon is another of too many with a history of long-term sexual abuse, physical abuse and gross neglect. Her mother was complicit in the abuse. What is glaringly absent in her history is that she never abused alcohol or drugs that are often contributing factors to successful suicides.

Although Sonja's last admission was primarily for depression and suicidal ideation, she was supported in maintaining her nutrition. In retrospect, this was likely a mistake. The very last thing she said to me before going out on pass was that she could not stand how fat she felt. I believe that, on this particular day, her fear of being fat was the primary triggering factor for her suicide. She should have been told to not worry about refeeding at this time and given permission to use the eating disorder as a temporary lifeline as she probably had done in the past. Two days earlier, in front of the nursing station, she asked if she could hug me. This hug was possibly her way of saying goodbye having already decided she was going to end her life.

During her last admission, she was started for the first time on the antidepressant fluoxetine. It is well known that depressed individuals who's moods lift due to taking antidepressants may attain the mental wherewithal to actually carry out a suicide. When in the more severe depressed state, individuals may not have the motivation or mental agility to organize a viable suicidal plan. In recent years, selective serotonin reuptake inhibitors have required warnings that suicidal tendencies may increase.

Lesson Points

- Ward staff cannot be too diligent in observing and protecting the suicidal individual. However, staff are often too busy to implement minute to minute watches for clients.
- Suicidal patients are remarkably resourceful when wanting to carry out suicide while hospitalized. Sharon found a detachable stereo cord in the quiet room she could have very easily used to hang herself.
- When an individual expresses suicidal ideation, especially connected to self body image loathing, think about putting the eating disorder directives on hold.
- For those with eating disorders who are suicidal, ask what the eating disorder means to them in regard to helping to keep them alive. It may be the only thing they feel is keeping them alive. It may be their lifeline when nothing else is.

Summary

Of those who successfully suicide, many have a long standing history of severe depression, multiple suicide attempts, as well as drug and alcohol abuse. Regretted sexual experiences including sexual assault are too commonly an associated factor as well. No matter how closely monitored suicidal individuals are, there inevitably will be windows of opportunity for them to take their life if they are so driven. Only a few minutes are required. Hospital admissions are no guarantee of safety.

Chapter 3

Critical Medical Conditions in Eating Disorders

The many stories mentioned throughout the book provide an inside look at what are largely real-life clinical situations. The medical risks highlighted in these stories were selected to help bring a heightened awareness of potential critical events. Chapter 4, *Eating Disorder Behaviors,* also addresses several medical risks. This chapter, *Critical Medical Conditions in Eating Disorders,* narrows in on select critical and lethal medical risks.

In-depth descriptions of the *Medical Complications of Eating Disorders*[1–3] and *The Medical Management of Eating Disorders*[1,4], can be found elsewhere in the literature.

Lethality

Lethal medical conditions in those with eating disorders mostly center around the heart. The heart is the inevitable end organ targeted by pathologies from several sources leading to death. The function of clinicians is to get in the way of or interfere with any and all potential causes of cardiac demise. Less than fatal sources of medical crises can affect a range of organs and systems and requires a broad understanding of medical risk.

Although critical medical risks are described under separate headings, many body systems are typically interlinked to create medical environments that lead to lethality. Yes, some will die of an inherent cardiac pathology that has not been influenced by other systemic etiologies such as starvation, metabolic irregularities, or other disturbances. However, those with eating disorders who starve, experience significant weight loss as well as engage in purging and other eating disorder behaviors will more likely adopt multisystem contributors to risk. The following focuses on the most critical and lethal contributors to medical crises.

Statistics and More Damn Lies

When attempting to find reliable sources for material regarding the medical complications of eating disorders, I used some of the most respected medical

DOI: 10.4324/9781003053088-3

review search engines. Many of the review articles I found had been updated as recently as three to four months previously. What I discovered, however, was that several of the original articles referenced to were decades old. It turns out that there is a paucity of truly current original research data. This brings to light a few observations.

There are a number of reasons to take the bulk of research articles with a grain of salt.

- The *Diagnostic and Statistical Manual for Mental Disorders* classifications for eating disorders has been updated 2–3 times since many papers have been written. Therefore, what had been defined as an eating disorder 25 years ago does not apply to today's classifications.
- Many studies were flawed due to small patient samples and faulty research methods.
- Much research has been reported on single case studies, therefore, not providing any statistical relevance.
- Several studies outright contradict each other.
- Laboratory testing and medical imaging technology have improved multifold over the years. Much older testing data can be incomplete and outdated by today's standards.
- Studies will have been and still are done on very select populations. To a large degree, data taken from major research centers sample from a more financially advantaged group. Many with eating disorders cannot afford hospital or residential based eating disorder programs and will not show up in statistics. Also, the majority of the literature comes from European and North American research centers thus disregarding sampling of those with eating disorders for most of the world's population. Eating disorders has been anecdotally reported as rampant in Asian countries such as Korea, Japan, and China. A colleague of mine visited a Beijing eating disorder program over thirty years ago. He said that eating disorders were, indeed, epidemic in China then.
- Those with eating disorders who haven't recovered as well as those who have recovered on their own, all without having been part of a formal research based program, will not have been documented and included in statistics.

Some statistics should be viewed as rough guidelines at best. Other statistics, for reasons mentioned above, should be glanced at but not relied upon. The most accurate data that I accept as relevant is from *single* case studies. The physical findings (height, weight, BMI, and physical examination) as well as blood and urine laboratory values, EKG, Holter monitor, echocardiogram, and other diagnostic determinants will largely be accurate especially from more recent studies. Clinical case reports stating "She was 5'5" and 74 lbs.

She ate less than 800 calories daily and vomited 8 times per day. Her heart rate was 27 bpm, blood pressure 80/45 and the EKG revealed several runs of ventricular tachycardia with periods of torsades de pointes and revealed a QTc interval of 580 msec. She died of sudden cardiac death." brings home the critical nature of eating disorders. Generalizing statements especially from review articles that report, as an example, "Those with eating disorders may experience bradycardia, ventricular dysrhythmias, demonstrate a prolonged QTc interval and have a BMI less than 17.5 may die of sudden cardiac death" do not have as much impact.

Cardiovascular Risks

The heart carries the highest risk to the cardiovascular system for those with eating disorders. There are, however, non-cardiac sources of risk that could lead to critical outcomes.

Cardiac Risks

The primary cardiac risks for those with eating disorders include:

- Mitral valve prolapse
- Other cardiac anomalies
- Prolonged QT syndrome
- Torsades de pointes
- Ventricular dysrhythmias
- Purkinje fiber disease
- Cardiomyopathy
- Heart rate variability abnormalities

Although these cardiac risk factors are listed separately, they very much can coexist. As an example, *mitral valve prolapse* (MVP) can be associated with several or even *all* of these other risks simultaneously making MVP a major threat for those with anorexia nervosa.

Other Cardiovascular Risks

Serious non-cardiac cardiovascular risks include:

- Disseminated intravascular coagulation (DIC)
- Vasoconstriction
- Cerebral emboli
- Superior mesenteric artery syndrome
- Esophageal or stomach renting leading to exsanguination

Cardiovascular Effects of Eating Disorders[5]

Eating disorders can have devastating consequences on multiple organ systems due to the state of starvation. The cardiovascular effects of anorexia nervosa have been well studied over the years. Some studies have cited the prolongation of the QT interval as the dominant trigger for cardiac arrhythmia and sudden death in this patient population. However, one meta-analysis found that the QTc interval in patients with anorexia nervosa was within normal range but significantly longer than in controls. Another important cardiovascular complication is the reduction of cardiac mass. Structural studies based mainly on ultrasound have shown a decrease in left ventricular mass, stroke volume, and cardiac output. One study found that women with anorexia nervosa have a significantly higher incidence of bradycardia, hypotension, mitral valve prolapse, decreased left ventricular mass, lower cardiac output, and lower cardiac index. The cause of these changes, in part, is still unknown. It has been postulated to be due to decreased preload, which leads to atrophy of cardiac muscle. Cardiac tamponade secondary to massive pericardial effusion has also been described recently.

Mitral Valve Prolapse

Mitral valve prolapse (MVP) is truly the mother ship of potential medical demise in those with eating disorders. Its capacity for both overt and occult medical risks needs to be clearly understood and anticipated.

Mitral valve prolapse is a cardiac anomaly that may carry significant lethal potential. Lethality is not just inherent in the anatomical irregularities of the mitral value unit (leaflets, chordae tendineae, annulus, and papillary muscle) but also in other etiologies that can accompany MVP. These include dysrhythmias such as ventricular tachycardia, other ventricular dysrhythmias as well as torsades de pointes, that are associated with sudden cardiac death. Other cardiac anomalies may coexist.

Atypical and non-anginal chest pain is the most common symptom attributed to mitral valve prolapse. Other manifestations may include palpitations, dyspnea, exercise intolerance, dizziness, or syncope and panic as well as anxiety disorders. Any combination of these symptoms and signs plus the typical auscultatory features of MVP have been defined as the *mitral valve prolapse syndrome*[6].

Definition of MVP

Definitions for MVP have changed over time. The diagnosis was typically based on clinical examination (auscultation) findings and echocardiogram derived criteria. The imaging definition for MVP is billowing of any portion of the mitral leaflets greater than or equal to 2 mm above the annular plane in a long-axis view. Prolapse of the mitral valve is defined as an abnormal systolic displacement of one or both leaflets into the left atrium (systolic billowing) due to a disruption or elongation of the leaflets, chordae, or papillary muscles[7].

Potential Mitral Valve Prolapse Risks

Mitral valve prolapse is a remarkably complicated condition. There are multiple variations of anatomical and mechanical pathology that can make up an individual's version of MVP[8]. Associated arrythmogenesis elevates risk. Dysrhythmias associated with MVP can vary in kind, regularity, severity, and lethality and are often unpredictable. Rhythmic variants may appear for the first time having evolved from previously occult potential. Aberrant electrical pathways may not express themselves until new stressors trigger them.

Mitral valve prolapse does not just exist as a static entity. Signs, symptoms, and valve unit function have the potential to become worse depending on genetics, cardiac structural changes, workload as well as aggravating non-MVP factors. Many can live with MVP without need for treatments such as medications, a pacemaker or defibrillator as well as surgery. For others, pathology can worsen requiring intervention. Sometimes death is the ultimate outcome.

The Mitral Valve Unit

The mitral valve consists of four basic structures namely the leaflets, papillary muscle, chordae tendinae, and annulus. Each of the mitral valve structures can be faulty by themselves but often exist in combination with other dysfunctional structures in the mitral valve unit.

Left Ventricle and Atrium

Compounding mitral valve dysfunction may be other cardiac pathology especially involving the *left atrium* and *left ventricle*. Shrinkage of the heart muscle including the atria and ventricles changes the relative structural architecture and function of the mitral value unit. The papillary muscle which is attached near the base of the left ventricle can allow the chordae tendinae to extend further causing the mitral leaflets to balloon into the atrium resulting in prolapse. This results in a misalignment of the leaflets with the annulus. Mitral regurgitation can result.

Ventricular Arrhythmias

There is evidence that the most common site of premature ventricular contraction (PVC) origin in those with MVP is the inferobasal left ventricular wall. This may be due to left ventricular myocardial scarring being the cause of electrical instability[8]. This scarring was discovered in 88% of young sudden cardiac death (SCD) victims with MVP. There is also evidence that there are papillary muscle-based PVCs. Diseased Purkinje tissue may be a source of PVCs. Although ventricular and other arrhythmias may be associated with MPV, they may exist without the presence of MVP.

Arrhythmic Complications of MVP[9]

There are various dysrhythmias associated with MVP. These include ventricular premature beats, premature atrial complexes, complex ventricular ectopy, paroxysmal supraventricular tachycarda, and ventricular fibrillation.

Arrhythmias may be more common in those with MVP who develop mitral regurgitation (MR). Moderate to severe MR is an independent predictor of ventricular as well as atrial arrhythmias.

Nonarrythmic Complications of MVP[10]

Complications of MVP that are not arrhythmic include:

• Mitral regurgitation
• Heart failure
• Infective endocarditis
• Cerebrovascular accidents

The most significant risk factors for mortality are the presence of moderate to severe mitral regurgitation and a left ventricular ejection fraction less than 50%.

Mitral Valve Prolapse and Sudden Cardiac Death

The mitral valve prolapse clinical presentation may range from a benign course to a catastrophic outcome such as sudden cardiac death. High-risk markers of MVP may include inverted or biphasic T waves, QT dispersions, QT prolongation, and premature ventricular contractions although there is some controversy regarding this. These originate from the left ventricular outflow tract and papillary muscles[11]. Morphofunctional characteristics of SCD are leaflet thickness of 5 mm or greater, mitral annulus disjunction, paradoxical systolic increase of the mitral annulus diameter, increased tissue Doppler velocity of the mitral annulus and higher mechanical dispersion on echocardiography and fibrosis observed on cardiac magnetic resonance imaging. Some newer markers identified are mechanical dispersion, myocardial work index, and postsystolic shortening but will need further research to validate relevance.

Sudden cardiac death in those with mitral valve prolapse is usually due to ventricular fibrillation[9]. MVP is the only cardiac abnormality found in 8–16%

of those with refractory ventricular tachycardia. On the other hand, both SCD and ventricular tachycardia can occur in patients without apparent structural heart disease.

The incidence of SCD in patients with MVP is not clearly established. One estimate of the risk of SCD in those with MVP without mitral regurgitation was 1.9 per 10,000 patients per year. The risk was estimated to be 50 to 100 times higher (0.9% to 1.9%) per year if significant mitral regurgitation is present.

The following factors may suggest an association between MVP and increased risk of SCD. These include:

- A history of syncope or near syncope
- Symptoms such as palpitations, chest pain and dyspnea
- Prolonged QT interval or inferolateral repolarization abnormalities
- Frequent or complex ventricular premature beats
- Prolapse of both the anterior and posterior mitral valve leaflets
- Hemodynamically significant mitral regurgitation
- Flail mitral leaflet

Proposed pathophysiologic mechanisms for SCD include fibrosis in the papillary muscles and inferobasal wall of the left ventricle, mitral annular disjunction, and systolic curling of the mitral leaflet. Premature ventricular complexes arising from the Purkinje tissue may be a trigger for ventricular fibrillation. Prior cardiac arrest or sustained ventricular tachycardia are strong predictors of SCD.

Mitral Valve Prolapse and Anorexia Nervosa

Mitral valve prolapse, by itself, can lead to serious health risks including sudden death. When combined in an individual with anorexia nervosa, risk can compound multifold. Significant weight loss in someone with anorexia nervosa who has never had an MVP previously can result in an MVP due to the anatomical alterations of the heart secondary to cardiac shrinkage, especially of the left ventricle, resulting in mitral valve disjunction with the annulus.

Anorexia nervosa can bring added risks to those already inherent in a patient with MVP such as:

- Metabolic abnormalities including mineral and electrolyte deficiencies
- General muscle wasting as well as wasting of the heart muscle mass involving the atria, ventricles and papillary muscles
- Physical stress, such as exercise, and psychological stress that can trigger ventricular dysrhythmias

- Further excitation or triggering potential of existing cardiac electrical irregularities already associated with MVP
- "Awakening" of occult or silent aberrant electrical pathology not yet expressed along with MVP

I recommend any individual with an eating disorder, regardless of whether they have bulimia or anorexia nervosa, who experiences palpitations or presents with the most minor of murmurs to have a thorough cardiac investigation early on in their contact with medical professionals. Waiting for signs and symptoms to get worse before taking the possibility of cardiac risks more seriously could be too late. Sudden cardiac death can occur without preceding overt clinical signs or threatening medical investigations.

Sudden Death in Eating Disorders[12]

Preventing *sudden death* in those with eating disorders is the prime focus for clinicians. We are all familiar with *sudden cardiac death* as the ultimate risk factor but there are non-cardiac sources of sudden death as well.

Sudden death has been defined as the abrupt and unexpected occurrence of fatality for which no satisfactory explanation of the cause can be ascertained. Although sudden deaths are often assumed to be of cardiac origin there is no way to confirm this with autopsy[1]. Regardless, research seems to support the main causes of sudden death in eating disorders are those related to cardiovascular complications.

A preventable cause of sudden death is the *refeeding syndrome*. This is an iatrogenic created lethal consequence of renourishing.

Standardized *mortality ratios* for anorexia nervosa vary from 1.36% to 20% and for bulimia, 1% to 3%.

Cardiovascular Complications and Sudden Death[12]

At least one-third of all deaths in patients with anorexia nervosa are estimated to be due to cardiac causes, mainly sudden death. Cardiovascular complication are common and they have been reported in up to 80% of the cases. Up to 10% of these complications were mainly bradycardia, hypotension, arrhythmias, repolarization abnormalities and sudden death. Food restriction can lead to increased vagal tone, bradycardia, orthostatic hypotension, syncope, arrhythmias, congestive heart failure, and sudden death[11].

With respect to QT abnormalities, QT interval is a measure of myocardial repolarization and its increased length is associated with life-threatening ventricular tachycardia. Therefore, a prolonged QT interval is a biomarker for ventricular tachyarrhythmia and a risk factor for sudden death. Sudden death in anorexia nervosa, like sudden death in liquid-protein dieting, might result from ventricular tachyarrhythmia related to QT interval prolongation.

The QT interval seems to have a poor predictive value for the recognition of patients who are at particular risk of sudden death. Only QT intervals greater than 600 milliseconds are clearly associated with significant risk of sudden death but few with eating disorders have such long QT intervals.

Considering the QT dispersion, an increase of the QT interval dispersion represents regional differences in myocardial excitability recovery and may lead to an increased arrhythmogenic substrate, with a higher risk of clinically significant ventricular arrhythmia and sudden death. Both prolonged QT interval and increased QT interval dispersion tend to normalize after re-feeding, along with heart rate and heart rate variability.

Those with eating disorders may show varying degrees of dehydration; sodium and chloride depletion, particularly in patients who vomit; potassium deficiency (in those who abuse laxatives); and weaknesses of chloride, sodium, and potassium in patients with diuretics, with different depletions depending on the substance used.[17] In the case of hypokalemia, repolarization abnormalities (prolonged and depressed QT interval and decreased height of the T-wave) are usually found. Cardiac or respiratory arrest is the most frequent cause of sudden death. T-wave flattening or inversion is present with potassium levels of 3.0–3.8 mEq/L (mmol/L) and a long QT interval, prominent U-wave, depression of the ST segment, and ventricular extrasystoles can be found with potassium levels of 2.3–3.0 mEq/L. Of particular interest is that torsades de pointes and ventricular fibrillation may be present with potassium levels less than 2.3 mEq/L. QTc prolongation and ventricular arrhythmia may develop in the setting of severe hypokalemia, exposing patients to high risk of a sudden cardiac event.[18]

Tako tsubo syndrome (apical ballooning syndrome) is a reversible cardiomyopathy triggered by acute emotional or physical stress that precedes it. As a result, cardiogenic shock and ventricular arrhythmias may cause death. The syndrome may follow hypoglycemia (which increases plasma catecholamine levels) have been described in anorectic patients. As well in a single case, an individual experienced several syncopal events due to recurrent episodes of torsades de pointes. The combination of tako tsubo caridomopathy associated with QT prolongation as well as possibly an increase of QT dispersion in someone with anorexia nervosa makes prognosis more severe.

Besides QT abnormalities, other causes of death have been described. Some unexpected autopsy findings have been reported including multiple bilateral pulmonary thromboembolisms and bilateral calf vein thrombosis. A 39 year-old woman with longstanding anorexia nervosa suffered a myocardial infarction of the inferior wall during refeeding. Anorexia nervosa does not "protect" against coronary atherosclerosis and some cases of sudden death may be related to myocardial ischemia. Lipofuscin accumulation in the myocardium has been reported.[24] Another possible mechanism of cardiovascular mortality and sudden death among those with eating disorders is the alteration in sympathovagal balance and an increased vagal tone.

Hypoglycemia and Sudden Death [12]

Hypoglycemia is well known in starvation including those with anorexia nervosa. Severe hypoglycemia in anorexia nervosa may occur without symptoms. Hypoglycemic coma is a complication in anorexia nervosa reflecting severe malnutrition indicating a poor and possibly fatal prognosis. Sudden death related to hypoglycemia has been reported in eating disorder patients, usually associated with other complications such as pulmonary edema, cerebral hemorrhage or coincident with acute exacerbation of liver injury induced by oral intake of nutrients.

Some etiological factors responsible for hypoglycemia can include excessive exercise, depletion of glycogen, gluconeogenesis failure as well as disturbances in glucagon secretion. Those with uncontroled IDDM are at particular risk.

Asphyxia, Gastric Dilatation, and Gastric Rupture [12]

Polyphagia has been reported to result in death due to asphyxiation. A sudden subdiaphragmatic viscus expansion with resultant lung volume displacement and impediment of venous return from the lower half of the body and infraglottic asphyxia have been reported as the main causes of death. Diaphragmatic contractility can be depressed in severely malnourished patients. This may cause acute respiratory distress and sudden death. Refeeding early enough can reverse these risks.

Eating disorders usually cause gastrointestinal disturbances, such as decreased gastric motility and delayed gastric emptying, which may rarely lead to acute gastric dilatation. Acute gastric dilatation can result in gastric necrosis, perforation, shock, and death. There are different causes of acute gastric distension (refeeding after starvation, diabetes mellitus, tumors, gastric volvulus, gastroduodenal tuberculosis, gastroduodenal Crohn's disease as examples). Approximately 60% of those with eating disorders will have gastric dysmotility and are at increased risk for acute gastric dilation due to decreased gastric motility, increased gastric capacity, and decreased gastric emptying. Gastric dilatation has been associated with *superior mesenteric* artery syndrome and acute *pancreatitis*.

Emetics [12]

Use of the emetic, *Ipecac*, can result in irreversible and potentially fatal cardiomyopathies. Death can result from cardiac origin such as myocarditis with arrhythmias. Myositis, gastroesophageal rupture, and metabolic abnormalities are other causes of death. Other substances used as emetics such as salt, gasoline and others bring their own risks.

Sepsis[12]

Postmortem has revealed *pneumonia* and *sepsis* on an individual with anorexia nervosa. Also noted was chronic interstitial nephritis, proximal tubular swelling, and diffuse glomerular sclerosis suggesting chronic glomerular injury. With regard to renal function, acute renal failure induced by the presence of rhabdomyolysis has been reported to have been caused by refeeding-induced hypophosphatemia. Prolonged electrolyte disturbances in anorexia nervosa, catabolism, and insufficient immunity are the main factors for developing an acute inflammation, as well as other complications such as cardiorespiratory failure, nosocomial infection, and sepsis with multiple organ failure.

Brain and Spinal Cord Findings at Postmortem[12]

It was noted in a patient who died of acute anorexia nervosa revealed a slim neuron type with one extremely long basal dendritic field. Reduction of spine morphology and reduction in spine density were noted.

Refeeding Syndrome[15–19]

The *refeeding syndrome* may be defined as the potentially fatal shift in fluids and electrolytes that may occur in starved individuals receiving renourishment. These shifts result from hormonal and metabolic changes. The primary biochemical feature of refeeding syndrome is hypophosphatemia as well as hypokalemia and hypomagnesemia[13]. The change to anabolism, which occurs during refeeding, causes an increase in insulin secretin and, consequently, potassium is taken into cells. As a result, disturbances in the electrochemical membrane potential can result in arrhythmias and cardiac arrest[13]. Hypomagnesemia also affects membrane potential leading to cardiac complications. Beside the changes in potassium and magnesium levels, in refeeding syndrome phosphous depletion occurs, which in turn leads to widespread dysfunction of cellular processes affecting almost every physiological system. Moreover, the introduction of *carbohydrates* to a diet leads to a rapid decrease in renal excretion of sodium and water. In this environment, patients may rapidly develop fluid overload with congestive cardiac failure pulmonary edema and cardiac arrhythmia[13,14].

The *refeeding syndrome* is a much talked about and somewhat feared consequence in the treatment of those with eating disorders. It also is shrouded in a degree of mystery. Although as clinicians we feel we understand what it is, there is no one definitive criteria to define it and is an extremely complicated condition to understand fully. It is, however, a potentially lethal result of poorly managed refeeding. Documentation of events that were likely the refeeding syndrome go back hundreds of years.

My wife's uncle was part of the original British and Canadian troops that liberated the Bergen-Belsen Nazi concentration camp in Germany, April 15, 1945. This camp is most famous for being the place where Anne Frank died. He said that the liberating soldiers would reach into their food kit packs, and generously give the emaciated prisoners their food rations. The prisoners would drop dead right in front of them. This kind of witnessed sudden death experience had been observed by many other soldiers who had done the same thing. Although deaths were initially suspected of being caused by a "digestive problem," it is now suspected that prisoners died of the refeeding syndrome. The scariest part about this story is how fast the prisoners died, that is, right during the act of eating. What could have added to the risk of sudden death is that many of the prisoners were ill with typhoid fever, typhus, and tuberculosis. Catastrophic outcomes for renourishing those with eating disorders should not in any way be underestimated.

Years ago I attended a four-day international conference on eating disorders in New York City. There were about 800 attendees. On the Friday, we were given the evening off to explore the wonders of the city. Coincidently, a documentary on Ancel Keys was being shown that same evening in the conference center. What conference member is going to want to attend a potentially very dry documentary on a Friday night in New York City? Well, over 300 individuals did. What I had not been aware of is that eating disorder researchers and clinicians around the world considered the Minnesota Starvation Experiment, conducted by the physiologist Ancel Keys in 1944 to1945, a cornerstone look into understanding starvation, a major component in anorexia nervosa. Psychological and medical parameters were assessed. Prior to the starvation experiment Ancel Keys had been commissioned by the US Army, in 1941, to develop rations for troops in combat called K-rations.

Minnesota Starvation Experiment[20]

At the University of Minnesota, this experiment was designed to study the physiological and psychological effects of severe and prolonged starvation as well as the subsequent effectiveness of renourishment strategies. The impetus for the study came with the fear of anticipated famine in Europe and Asia at the end of World War II and how to deal with its consequences.

Thirty-six Caucasian men were chosen from a pool of conscientious objectors. Prior to the starvation phase of the study, they were fed 3200 calories daily. They would then be expected to lose 25% of their weight at a rate of 2.5 lbs a week. They were given about 1570 calories daily. They were also expected to walk 22 miles a week, work several hours a day in a lab and spend education time. As well, they were expected to keep a diary. Their nutrition consisted of bread, potatoes, cereal, turnip and cabbage, a diet mimicking available affordable food consumed in Europe at the time. All subjects were assessed to be healthy both physically and psychologically. Following the period of starvation, they would be exposed to various rehabilitation diets.

Note that 1570 calories was considered *severe starvation* food restriction for this study. We see those with eating disorders eating 200, 100, and 50 calories daily plus possibly vomiting and over-exercising as well. This should be a reminder of how extreme starvation can become and that working with those with eating disorders is not for the faint of heart.

Aside from emaciation, subjects experienced low temperature, heart rate, and blood pressure, felt cold and tired, had muscle wasting and were weak. All of this information we would intuitively expect from severe starvation. A large government study did not have to be conducted to gather this particular information. Although the physical findings of these scientific studies have relevance, the psychological findings were a major revelation.

The Psychological Expression of Starvation

The following are some signs and symptoms of severe starvation. Note the large number of psychological expressions.

- Depression
- Anxiety
- Social withdrawal
- Irritability
- Restlessness
- Apathy and lack of joy
- Being uncooperative
- Poor concentration
- Impulsivity
- Irrational thoughts
- Forgetfulness
- Short temper
- Lashing out
- Poor insight
- Mental fatigue
- Mood swings
- Difficulty sleeping
- Preoccupation with food
- Emotional instability
- Obsessive thoughts and behaviors
- Loss of sense of humor
- Hopelessness and helplessness
- Nihilism
- Paranoia
- Psychosis

Deanna's Story

Deanna was an 18 year-old young woman admitted to an adult eating disorder program with anorexia nervosa. She was 5 feet 7 inches and 96 lbs having lost 16 lbs in the last few weeks. She lost 45 lbs over the last year due to restricting, vomiting, and exercise compulsion. She presented with multiple psychological problems that greatly interfered with treatment for the eating disorder, including refeeding.

It was clear upon admission that she was very depressed. She was restless, short tempered, and would lash out. She would isolate in her room avoiding staff and family but would roam the ward at night not able to sleep. She would not cooperate with staff regarding attending groups or nutrition protocols. Although she refused to eat much of anything, she would pick at food during meals and snacks for long periods of time. She was obsessed with food, constantly focused on it. She talked as if she had no future, was not good at anything, and her lot in life was hopeless. She was totally unmotivated to engage. She seemed paranoid that staff had been slipping her extra calories into her food. She displayed all or nothing thinking, refusing to consider other treatment options. She also perseverated about having not visited her grandmother enough.

Discussion

Deanna showed psychological symptoms of depression, agitation, restlessness, chronic insomnia, paranoia, food obsession, social withdrawal, obsessive-compulsive disorder, hopelessness, and nihilism. These symptoms were quite extreme.

A few decades ago Deanna would have likely been given antidepressants, sedatives, and possibly antipsychotic medications. She would have been labeled with borderline personality disorder or possibly bipolar spectrum disorder. A diagnosis of borderline personality disorder would likely have excluded her from treatment for her eating disorder and would have been discharged from the hospital as soon as possible. This would be because of a belief by staff that she would habituate to the ward and then make efforts to avoid being discharged. Electroconvulsive therapy might have been considered as well in order to treat the unrelenting depression.

With the Minnesota Starvation Experiment findings becoming more recognized in the clinical eating disorder world, it has become more evident that *all* of the psychological symptoms Deanna had been exhibiting could easily have been symptoms of starvation, not endogenous mental illness. All of these symptoms could improve and clear with full renourishment. The focus of treatment for her psychological presentation should be restoring nutrition and correcting any medical irregularities. Those symptoms not necessarily attributable to starvation may persist after renourishing indicating a non-starvation etiology and, therefore, further treatment options may need to be considered.

Lesson Points

- A multitude of serious psychological symptoms can present with starvation.
- The "medicine" for these symptoms is food.
- Psychological symptoms that could evolve from starvation may not be starvation-induced.
- If psychological symptoms predate starvation, then observe whether they worsen with starvation. Preexisting depression, anxiety, obsessive-compulsive traits, paranoia, and insomnia may worsen with starvation.
- Psychotropic medications may not work as expected in those who are starved. Brain chemistry may be significantly altered due to starvation.

Starvation Can Lead To Lasting Physiological and Psychological Change

After one recovers from starvation many medical and psychological signs and symptoms will resolve. Some may, however, persist. Starvation can be viewed as a kind of trauma or assault on the body. Any system can be affected. Many systems may be affected concurrently or possibly in a serial temporal order. Permanent damage to various organs will result from severe and prolonged exposure to starvation. Shorter exposure might put the individual at high risk at the moment but the body would likely "spring back" to health before lasting damage occurred. However, there can be no predicting as to what would be considered too prolonged exposure to starvation and, therefore, too late for recovery.

If the heart has been starved long enough, it can become permanently damaged and full recovery will not be possible. The heart may recover enough to function adequately for years but it can weaken later in life and fail to keep someone alive. This is similar to what happens to skeletal muscle after someone acquires polio. After the initial exposure to the poliovirus, other muscles compensate for the affected paralyzed ones. These healthy muscles are, however, overcompensating and cannot sustain this for many years. They become weak later in life leading to the *post-polio syndrome*. Similarly, the heart of a chronically starved person with anorexia nervosa may be able to compensate for a few years then ultimately fail.

Prolonged starvation can have a serious effect on the brain. Radiographic imaging shows the brain can shrink and the ventricles expand. Neurological symptoms can arise as well as psychological ones.

Insulin-Dependent Diabetes Mellitus

There is little more terrifying for clinicians than trying to medically manage an individual who has an eating disorder and insulin-dependent diabetes mellitus (IDDM). For those who want to have good control of their diabetes yet have an active full-on eating disorder, good glucose control can be difficult. For others who refuse to take insulin, monitor their glucose levels as well as balance adequate nutrition and exercise, management of diabetes and an eating disorder can become a nightmare. Restricting food, binge eating, vomiting, and exercise compulsion play havoc with serum glucose levels. Some will not monitor glucose levels yet give themselves a guessed-at insulin dose. Diabetic coma or insulin-induced coma are very real lethal risks that can develop within minutes allowing for no immediate medical intervention. Studies have shown patients with weight loss related to insulin restriction, diabulimia, were 3.2 times more likely to die over an 11-year period and to die an average of 13 years younger than those who did not restrict insulin[21]. Consider those with IDDM and an eating disorder the most at risk individuals for lethal outcome. See *Withholding Insulin* in Chapter 4, *Eating Disorder Behaviors*.

Obstetric and Gynecologic Concerns Associated With Eating Disorders

Common obstetric and gynecologic complications for women with eating disorders include infertility, unplanned pregnancy, miscarriage, poor nutrition during pregnancy, having a baby with small head circumference, postpartum depression and anxiety, sexual dysfunction, and complications in the treatment of gynecologic cancers[22,23]. There are unique associations between eating disorder diagnoses, such as earlier cessation of breast-feeding in anorexia nervosa; increased polycystic ovarian syndrome in bulimia; and complications of obesity as a result of binge eating disorder.

Although women with anorexia nervosa do not appear to differ from the general population in the incidence of breast or female genital cancers, their risk of mortality from gynecologic cancers is twice as high as the general population (uterine and ovarian cancers) as indicated in one sample. This may be due to delay in diagnosis and treatment of gynecologic malignancies in individuals with anorexia nervosa and possibly decreased effectiveness of treatments due to malnutrition. Some women with binge eating disorder may be at increased risk of developing endometrial cancer as obese women are at increased risk of endometrial cancers.

Please peruse the superb original articles listed below for in-depth discussions regarding given topics and a thorough collection of references.

References

1. Mehler P. Anorexia nervosa in adults and adolescents: Medical complications and their management. *UpToDate, Literature review current through*: Sep 2021.
2. Mitchel JE, et al. Bulimia nervosa and binge eating disorder in adults: Medical complications and their management. *UpToDate. Literature review current through*: Aug 2020.
3. Westmoreland P, et al. Medical complications of anorexia nervosa and bulimia. *The American Journal of Medicine*. 2016;**129**:30–37.
4. Birmingham CL and Treasure J. *Medical Management of Eating Disorders*. 3rd Edition. Cambridge University Press. July 2019.
5. Lamzabi L, Syed S, Reddy VB, Jain R, Harbhajanka A, and Arunkumar P. Myocardial changes in a patient with anorexia nervosa: a case report and review of literature. *American Journal of Clinical Pathology* 2015;**143**:734–737. 10.1309/AJCP4PLFF1TTKENT
6. Sorrentino M. Mitral valve prolapse syndrome. *UpToDate*. Literature review current through: Oct 2021.
7. Pislaru S, et al. Definition and diagnosis of mitral valve prolapse. *UpToDate*. Literature review current through: Oct 2021.
8. Basso C, et al. Mitral valve prolapse, ventricular arrhythmias, and sudden death. *Circulation*. 2019:**140**:952–964.
9. Sorrentino MJ. Arrhythmic complications of mitral valve prolapse. *UpToDate*. Literature review current through: Oct 2021.
10. Pislaru S, et al. Arrhythmic complications of mitral valve prolapse. *UpToDate*. Literature review current through: Oct 2021.
11. Muthukumar L, et al. Association between malignant mitral valve prolapse and sudden cardiac death. *JAMA Cardiol*. 2020;**5**(9):1053–1056. 10.1001/jamacardio.2020.1412
12. Jauregui-Garrido B, et al. Sudden death in eating disorders. *Vascular Health Risk Manag*. 2012;**8**:91–98. Published online 2012 Feb 15. Doi:10.2147/VHRM.S28652 https://www.ncbi.nlm.nih.gov/pmc/articles/PMC3292410/
13. Mehanna HM, et al. Refeeding syndrome: what it is and how to prevent and treat it. *BMJ*. 2008;**336**(7569):1495–1498.
14. Veverbrants E, et al. Effects of fasting and refeeding. I. Studies on sodium, potassium and water excretion on a constant electrolyte and fluid intake. *J Clin Endocrinol Metab*. 1969;**29**(1):55–62.
15. Crook MA, et al. The Importance of the refeeding syndrome. *Nutrition*. 2001;**17**: 632–637.
16. Hisham M. Mehanna, et al. Refeeding syndrome: what it is, and how to prevent and treat it. *BMJ*. 2008;**336**(7659):1495–1498. doi: 10.1136/bmj.a301, www.ncbi.nlm.nih.gov/pmc/articles/PMC2440847/
17. Refeeding Syndrome and Sudden Death. Brian Dunning. Skeptoid Podcast #672. April 23, 2019. Podcast transcript.
18. Refeeding syndrome is underdiagnosed and under treated, but treatable. Stephen D Hearing. *BMJ* 2004;**328**(7445):908–909. doi:10.1136/bmj/328.7445908

19. Anorexia nervosa in adults and adolescents: The refeeding syndrome. Philip Mehler, MD. www.uptotdate.com ©2020 UpToDate
20. Keys A, Brozek J, Henschel A, Mickelsen O, and Taylor HA. *The Biology of Human Starvation* (2 Volumes), University of Minnesota Press, 1950.
21. http://nationaleatingdisorders.org/diabulimia-5
22. Kimmel MC, et al. Obstetric and gynecologic problems associated with eating disorders. *Int. J. Eat. Disord.* 2015;**49**:(3)260–275. 10.1002/eat.22483
23. Ward V. Eating Disorders in pregnancy. *BJM.* 2008 Jan 12;**336**(7635):9396. doi:10.1136/bmj.39393.689595.BE

Chapter 4

Eating Disorder Behaviors

The utilization of *eating disorder behaviors* is a major cause of medical risk and crisis for those with eating disorders. *All* eating disorder specific medical risks stem from these behaviors. Enquiring with great accuracy regarding a client's use of these behaviors is crucial in diverting potential risks. We, therefore, need to have a working knowledge of body image control behaviors employed by those with eating disorders.

An *eating disorder behavior* is any behavior that is used for any eating disorder purpose. The ultimate goal for implementing a given eating disorder behavior is to assist in controlling weight, body shape, and body image. They also may serve to cope with an array of emotions whether eating disorder related or otherwise.

The primary eating disorder behavior categories are:

- Purging Behaviors
- Calorie Burning and Metabolism Altering Behaviors
- Body Gauging Behaviors
- Binge Eating and Related Behaviors
- Restricting Eating Behaviors
- False Information
- Organizing Behaviors
- Symptom Management Behaviors
- Surgery and Other Cosmetic Altering Methods
- Substance Use

Some behaviors obviously present as major medical risks while others are not as likely to do so. Because relative risks of each behavior have not been investigated to date, we need to be open to the possibility of *unknown risks* being in the mix. As mentioned elsewhere, the potential accumulated risk from each behavior when combined with others in use should be considered.

Since any of us will not be able to bring to the front of our minds all of the eating disorder behaviors listed here when we want to, use this section of the book as a reference for the future. More extensive coverage of this material is

DOI: 10.4324/9781003053088-4

available elsewhere[1]. Although quite a comprehensive compilation of these behaviors has been collected here, there will undoubtedly be others that have not been accounted for. Watch for them regardless.

The anticipated most dangerous eating disorder behaviors have been discussed in some depth.

Purging Behaviors

Vomiting, the use of laxatives, suppositories, enemas as well as *diuretics, breastfeeding, withholding insulin, phlebotomy,* and *rumination* are kinds of purging behaviors when used for body image control purposes.

Vomiting

Self-induced v*omiting* is a defining behavior for bulimia nervosa and commonly used in anorexia nervosa. It may also occur in *Other Specified Feeding or Eating Disorders.*

Reasons for Vomiting

Those with eating disorders may vomit for specific *eating disorder reasons*, for *non-eating disorder reasons* or both. Some individuals diagnosed with eating disorders may vomit but not for body image and weight control purposes. Leave the option open that these individuals may not, indeed, have an eating disorder but have been incorrectly diagnosed with one.

Eating Disorder Specific Reasons for Vomiting

- To lose weight, maintain weight, or prevent weight gain
- To control body image including body shape and body size

Non-Eating Disorder Specific Reasons for Vomiting

- To relieve abdominal pain or bloating
- To punish ones self for overeating
- To relieve stress
- To acquire or maintain a critical medical status to prevent discharge from hospital or prove the individual can take eating disorder behaviors to extremes
- A slow suicide
- To deal with remembrances of sexual assault
- To deal with guilt and shame
- To punish family
- To display a cry for help

- Because of a viral gastroenteritis, tuberculosis meningitis, brain tumor, malignancy, or hepatitis
- Because of other possible reasons

Methods of Inducing Vomiting

There are many ways of inducing vomiting. Some may be more dangerous than others, however, know that *all* forms of vomiting bring risk.

FINGERS

The most common method of inducing vomiting is the use of fingers. Any individual finger or combination of fingers may be utilized. Most will engage one particular finger or a specific couple of fingers routinely to induce vomiting and this will usually be adequate for the task. Other fingers may be added to hopefully increase stimulation of the gag reflex when the gag reflex becomes less effective. If using the index finger, for example, is not being effective enough on its own, the middle, ring finger as well as the little finger may be added. Be aware of increasing use of multiple fingers as this implies a diminishing or even total absence of the gag reflex. The declining effectiveness of the gag reflex can lead individuals to panic and introduce other methods of triggering vomiting that may, in turn, be more dangerous such as the use of emetics, spoons, spatulas or other implements. Be alerted to alternative behaviors to vomiting as these too may be dangerous. That is, other eating disorder behaviors may temporarily replace vomiting. As well, self-harm behaviors including suicide attempts may arise.

SPOONS, SPATULAS, AND OTHER UTENSILS

Aside from fingers, utensils may come into play to induce vomiting. These may be spoons, spatulas, chop sticks, tooth brushes, or any other long, thin device that can reach to the back of the throat in an attempt to trigger the gag reflex.

Utensils will likely be chosen when fingers begin to fail. However, they may be chosen out of personal preference and not necessarily because of increased effectiveness. Some feel that the use of fingers is undesirable because fingers may be deemed dirty or it may be that individuals just don't like the idea of it. There is a kind of "yuck" factor for some.

Medical risks may include scratching of the oropharynx, damage to the vocal cords, or utensils becoming lodged in the throat. The handle of a spatula may snap off. Removal of the implement may have to take place in the ER. It is possible to suffocate from a lodged utensil.

Aside from spoons and spatulas, items may be dangled down the throat with a string to induce vomiting. A paper click or other objects may be used.

EMETICS

Emetics are substances that when ingested trigger vomiting. They do this by causing extreme nausea through gastric irritation or stimulation of the chemorecteptor trigger zone in the brain. They tend to be utilized when attempting vomiting when other mechanisms fail. They may, of course, be a first line method preferred by some.

The most famous and likely most dangerous emetic was a commercial pharmaceutical called Ipecac. The active chemical was emetine. This was a particularly dangerous compound because it caused severe, violent stomach contractions that could lead to esophageal and gastric tears and ultimately serious and even fatal internal bleeding. Bleeding would be obvious when presenting through the mouth or occult when transported through the bowel. Frank rectal bleeding or melena stools could present. Emetine is a myotoxin and can cause dysrhythmias and cardiomyopathy. It has been fatal in small doses taken over time.

Salt is a common, inexpensive, and easily available substance when used as an emetic. Salt may be delivered by being dissolved in water and then drunk or undissolved when put on wet fingers or chop sticks then licked off. It causes severe nausea resulting in the drive to vomit. It too may be dangerous as it can cause extremely forceful vomiting urges and salt toxicity. Mustard can also be used as an emetic in powdered or liquid form.

Although salt and Ipecac have been the most popular emetics, be aware that *other* substances may be consumed with the hope of it acting as an emetic. These substances may be toxic. Floor cleaners including those that contain methanol or peroxide may be used. Drain cleaners that contain caustic substances can chemically burn the mouth and throat and, as well, are toxic. Gasoline is used as an emetic.

SPONTANEOUS VOMITING WITHOUT STIMULATING GAG REFLEX

Those with eating disorders who have become practiced in vomiting may become adept at vomiting spontaneously. That is, they are able to vomit at will without using fingers, utensils, or emetics. All some have to do is just bend over a garbage bin or toilet to make this happen.

INVOLUNTARY VOMITING

Some with eating disorders may vomit involuntarily possibly because they have developed an extremely low threshold for vomiting. This creates great anxiety as it may happen in any public setting. It may happen with eating lunch or dinner at home or in a restaurant when eating with others. It could happen at school or the workplace as well. Mental or visual images may trigger involuntary vomiting.

VOMITING WHILE SLEEPING OR UNCONSCIOUS

Some may vomit while sleeping or unconscious such as when, intoxicated. It also may occur while experiencing a spontaneous vasovagal event. There is a risk of choking on vomitus while sleeping or unconscious, leading to suffocation with resulting brain damage or death. Those who wake up vomiting from sleep find it deeply disturbing and are fearful of it happening again.

What Do Individuals Vomit?

We expect that those with eating disorders typically vomit food. They may also deliberately vomit other substances.

- Air
- Clear water
- Blood
- Bile
- Markers

Ending Vomiting Sessions – Endpoints

For every session of vomiting, individuals will end each session because of a specific reason. An obvious reason to stop vomiting is because it is believed that enough or possibly all stomach contacts have been expelled. Studies have shown that between 60% and 80% of stomach contents are removed due to vomiting. Some rely on what they feel is a more objective determination of emptying stomach contents by observing blood, bile, clear fluid, or markers return.

Physical symptoms including chest pain, palpitations, feeling dizzy or experiencing syncope may also be an indication to stop vomiting. These symptoms tend to bring fear.

Where Do Individuals Vomit?

Those with eating disorders can vomit virtually anywhere. They can vomit in any room in their own home, their parent's, friend's or partner's homes, at school, in their car, at work or onto the street from their car while stopped at an intersection. Individuals may vomit directly into different disposal devices or containers.

Typically, individuals vomit into toilets. They may, however, vomit into bathroom or kitchen sinks, shower drains, garbage cans, plastic or paper bags, plastic food containers, planters or flowerbeds. Some may vomit into napkins or tissues and place this in their pocket temporarily with the intension of disposing of it later. Some will vomit into plastic food containers, Styrofoam cups or bags for temporary storage.

When Individuals Can't Vomit

There are different reasons individuals are unable to vomit. Some are unable to vomit due to their gag reflex not being stimulated enough or at all. Other reasons can be that as someone has just binged but are then unable to vomit because a family member, partner or roommate has just returned home. Some are unable to vomit with ease depending on the type of food they have eaten. That is, some foods are easier to vomit than others.

As mentioned with regard to athletes who have injuries and can't exercise excessively, those who can't vomit at will panic and sometimes go to great lengths to compensate. Some may revert to using emetics when they normally would not. Severe restricting measures, exercising, and introducing other eating disorder behaviors to compensate for not being able to vomit may be engaged. Alcohol or drug use as well as suicidal ideation may ensue.

Medical Risks From Vomiting

Medical risks created from vomiting are likely to escalate because of the following.

(See *Increased Use of Eating Disorder Behaviors* in Chapter 1: *Introduction*)

Vomiting Frequency

Individuals who vomit to control body image and weight may vary the use of vomiting or maintain a routine, predictable pattern possibly deviating from this at times. Increasing the frequency of vomiting will likely increase medical risks.

When enquiring regarding vomiting frequency, we need to know whether this is on a monthly, weekly, or daily basis. Ask regarding why they have chosen the frequency they use and why it changes if it does.

Consumption Volume

Consumption volume may affect risk. Some who vomit may attempt to vomit very small food quantities of food such at a single cracker. Some will even attempt to vomit air from their stomachs having not eaten or drunk anything for a day or more. Some will binge eat on remarkably large quantities of food several times in a day. Binges of over 50,000 to 80,000 calories and more in a single day have been reported.

Medical risk may come from severe stretching of the stomach that in turn may cause it to rupture and lead to exsanguination. Vomiting large quantities of food quickly with great force and increased frequency may tear the cardia and esophagus.

Force of Vomiting

Some are able to vomit with little effort. Others may require more force with each attempt. The need for more force may come with a declining or absent gag reflex or having to vomit an inordinately large quantity of food quickly.

The *kinds of foods* also determine the ease or difficulty of vomiting. Foods that some find difficult to vomit may be easier for others. As an example, some find pasta difficult to vomit while others will chose pasta due to its ease of evacuating the stomach. Liquids tend to be easy to vomit while salads and breads may be difficult depending on the individual.

Number of Single Vomiting Events and Vomiting Sessions

The number of times one will vomit in a day can vary from zero to 80 times or more. When asking regarding how many times one vomits, we need to ask whether they mean *individual vomiting events* or *sessions of vomiting* where one will vomit a number of separate times during each session.

This distinction is very important. If one vomits three separate individual times in a day then medical risk is likely lower than if they vomit 15 times during *each* of three sessions – a total of 45 individual times daily.

Patterns of Vomiting

If individuals vomit in particular predictable patterns, determine what these are. Some patterns, as an example, may involve vomiting two sessions daily – once in the morning and once in the evening. Some may vomit after every time they eat. These patterns and others may be repeated predictably day after day. Some do not vomit in particular patterns and will vomit sporadically as triggered by random events. Enquire why one might deviate from their usual patterns.

Duration of Vomiting Events

Ask how long a vomiting session lasts and does it ever vary. If session times vary, determine the *range of time*. It's important to know why there are varying times.

Reasons to increase the duration of vomiting sessions are:

*   Binge food quantity consumed has been increased
*   Binge foods chosen are more difficult to vomit than others

- The individual fears not being able to rid enough stomach contents without more time to vomit
- The individual wishes to increase the percent of food removed from the stomach than is usually purged
- The gag reflex is declining in sensitivity and it is becoming harder to vomit
- The individual is in a vomiting "zone" where they wish to just take their time
- They are mentally and possibly physically tired and do not have the oomph to hurry a session
- They don't have access to vomiting aids such as fluids, utensils, or emetics to assist in the vomiting process
- They are inebriated
- They have multiple sclerosis
- Any other reason

Shifting Vomiting Endpoints

As mentioned earlier, individuals will end a session of vomiting for a particular reason. That is, they have a specific endpoint for which they will chose to stop. The reason or reasons chosen may be the same every time or, however, may shift in given situations. The changing of a selected endpoint may indicate difficulties in executing vomiting. As an example, one may typically use seeing blood at the end of a vomiting session as an indication to stop vomiting but then may choose to use the sight of bile or experience chest pain when blood cannot be visualized.

Toxicity

Another medical risk associated with vomiting is the toxicity of substances used to aid in vomiting.

Water is commonly used to help ease vomiting. It is consumed along with solid foods to assist making food more of a slurry which is easier to bring up. Water intoxication may be a consequence of this along with fluid loading used to decrease hunger. Brain edema is possible.

Some liquids may be used instead of water such as alcohol, cleaning solutions, and possibly others. Alcohol use may lead to intoxication and loss of consciousness during which individuals may choke on their own vomit. Cleaning solutions, including peroxide, are poisonous and could lead to death. As mentioned earlier, emetics, including salt, may be toxic.

Prevention of Medication Absorption

Any medication taken orally soon after ingestion, can be evacuated with vomiting. Those who vomit will be advised to take medications well before a session of vomiting or after anytime. The problem with this advice is medications may stay in the stomach hours after being taken. This is due to the *intestinal dysmotility syndrome.* Some say they vomit food that had been eaten 12 hours earlier. Gastric emptying ceases along with peristalsis. Some say that pills may be vomited still intact after several hours having not dissolved.

Some medications, if vomited, will not create any significant problems. However, those required to take oral potassium or magnesium tablets or the oral contraceptive pill could have serious consequences if these medications are purged. When prescribing medications, determine when they are usually taken and find out when vomiting will occur in relation to this. Enquire as to whether or not individuals vomit food or medications consumed hours earlier.

Because potassium and other mineral supplements are critical in keeping those prone to metabolic irregularities alive, liquid delivery systems may be advised assuming they will be absorbed faster than in pill form. Some tablets may be effectively dissolved in water then consumed. The only way to determine if medications in solid or liquid form have been absorbed efficiently is to determine if serum levels rise in response to oral intake. Intramuscular injections or intravenous delivery may be the best and only options for some medications.

Regarding the birth control pill, there are other excellent options for contraception. Intrauterine devices, the contraceptive patch, and Depo-Provera injects are highly effective. In a pinch, until another reliable contraceptive method is available, the pill may be taken vaginally where it will be absorbed effectively. Condoms along with spermicide are also an effective method. Amenorrhea resulting from weight loss, high level exercise or both is not a guarantee ovulation is not occurring.

Those who rely on oral medications such as anitcoagulants, antipsychotics, cardio-active medications as well as other important medications need to be medically monitored closely. Pregnant women who require antinauseants may need to use injectable delivery instead of oral.

Medical risks from vomiting may also include:

- Choking
- Aspiration and asphyxia
- Tearing of the esophagus and stomach
- Metabolic abnormalities
- Cardiac irregularities
- Bleeding from the nose, oropharynx, esophagus, stomach or rectum.

Choking

Choking is a risk when individuals vomit, especially when associated with binge eating. Choking may result from food or vomitus being inhaled during binging and vomiting sessions.

Aspiration and Asphyxiation

These can occur with inhalation of food or vomitus. There will be higher risk of this if an individual is inebriated and even more so if someone is unconscious. Someone who is in a great hurry may inadvertently lodge food in their trachea due to not being careful with binging and vomiting coordination. Someone who loses consciousness due to a vasovagal event may regurgitate food and then inhale vomitus therefore choking on this. Those who become unconscious will not have awareness of choking and suffocating.

Tearing of Esophagus and Stomach

Vomiting can cause tears in the esophagus, stomach or both. The likelihood of this happening will increase with the *volume of food* to be expelled, the *force* or *pressure* created with vomiting and the *rapidity* of each vomiting event.

The cardia is a functional structure located at bottom of the esophagus where it joins the stomach. At rest, the opening to the cardia is elongated and about the size of a dime. Forcing large quantities of food through this orifice over a second or two into the esophagus during vomiting can cause renting or tearing. Bleeding can be minor or lethal. Bleeding can be drained distally through the intestines, without evidence of any bleeding through the mouth. Exsanguination can occur silently.

Hyperability to vomit

When performing a pre-op assessment for someone going for surgery, I caution the anesthetist to be particularly alert to the possibility of unconscious, spontaneous vomiting post-operatively. I advise nursing staff to closely monitor post-op patients, watching for vomiting during recovery. I am particularly concerned for those having had jaw surgery during which their jaws have been wired shut.

Metabolic Abnormalities

Vomiting can lead to a whole range of metabolic abnormalities especially if there are other compounding etiologies. *Metabolic abnormalities* are mentioned in Chapter 3: *Critical Medical Conditions*.

Laxatives

Laxatives may be used on their own with the intention of losing weight. Weight loss occurs through *removal of stool* and possibly *fluids* in the form of diarrhea. It, of course, does not affect weight through adipose tissue reduction or affect lean body mass. Laxatives are sometimes used with the belief that food is transported through the small bowel so quickly that there is not enough time for nutrition absorption to be carried out. With the small bowel being about 9 to 16 feet long and digestive enzymes working rather quickly, food will likely be absorbed efficiently regardless of gut transit speed. However, some claim that they see undigested food in the toilet after laxative use. I would trust this reported observation from those that mention it.

Aside from the above purposes, laxatives are used by those with eating disorders for the purpose of stimulating bowel motion from a gut that has become slow. This slowness may be caused by the *intestinal dysmotility syndrome* resulting in lessening frequency of bowel movements and even constipation. The bowel can also slow down due to *bowel habituation* to laxatives and *poisoning* of the gut nerve plexuses from laxative use. The nerve plexuses can be destroyed resulting in permanently paralyzed gut muscle. The more individuals try to increase gut motility with laxatives, the more it resists and slows down. The bowel can become so slow that some report not being able to have a bowel movement for a week or two and develop hard constipated stool that requires the use of enemas along with laxatives. A tap water enema may need to be performed in a hospital out-patient unit.

Some may start with two tablets of laxatives infrequently in order to stimulate bowel movements successfully then eventually need to increase use to 30, 40 and 50 or more tablets daily to perform the same function. Laxative use can be a very expensive enterprise.

Laxative use can also result in the *malabsorption syndrome* due to destruction of the *villi* and *microvilli* of the small intestine. This will contribute to the inability of the bowel to absorb a large number of nutrients. Autoimmune causes of malabsorption must be considered when nutrition status is seriously compromised regardless of suspected eating disorder etiologies. Serious medical risk comes from electrolyte imbalances due to the loss of electrolytes in diarrheal stools. Diarrhea also contributes to dehydration. Electrolyte loss and dehydration from laxative use can compound the electrolyte loss and dehydration resulting from vomiting as well as restriction of food and fluids. While laxative use, vomiting and restricting behaviors individually may not create much risk, the accumulative effect of all three sets of behaviors can be extreme.

Laxatives may be used to deliberately cause serious medical problems such as metabolic irregularities, syncope as well as dysrhythmias. These medical conditions can be a goal in themselves. They indicate to the individual that they have gone to extreme enough measures to feel successful with their eating disorder efforts. Laxatives may be used exclusively for dealing with constipation alone without the intent of losing weight or creating medical problems.

Laxative use can create significant hygiene, logistical, and embarrassment concerns. To avoid others from thinking they are using the toilet, they may pass diarrhea stools down the shower drain. Transportation on public transit or in a car has to be timed so that there is as short a time period as possible to the next available toilet. Some will soil themselves accidently.

Laxatives come in different forms and brands. Some will be relatively harmless while others can be destructive.

- Bulk-forming agents
- Emolient agents (stool softeners)
- Lubricant agents
- Stimulant agents
- Hyperosmotic agents
- Saline laxative agents
- Miscellaneous: castor oil
- Serotonin agonists
- Chloride channel activators

Enemas

Enemas are liquids injected into the rectum with the intention of stimulating a bowel movement. Unlike laxatives, they only affect a small part of the large bowel, the rectum. It has no effect on absorption of food and will not create dehydration or electrolyte loss. If used in excess they can, however, cause *phosphate poisoning*. There are various kinds of commercial enemas on the market. Some may develop a psychological dependence on their use.

Suppositories

Similar to enemas, suppositories are inserted into the rectum to chemically trigger bowel movement. Suppositories are not likely to cause or aggravate medical concerns. Individuals can become psychologically dependent on them. There are different kinds of commercial suppositories that can be purchased from pharmacies.

Diuretics

Diuretics are chemicals that trigger water and salt excretion from the body. Diuretics may be obtained over the counter or by prescription. They may be delivered to the body orally, intramuscularly, or intravenously. Therapeutic uses for diuretics are to relieve edema caused from kidney failure and congestive heart failure, control blood pressure, relieve premenstrual symptoms, glaucoma, and other conditions.

Diuretics are used by those with eating disorders to aid in weight loss through diuresis. Water is a heavy substance so diuretics may be effective in weight loss at least temporarily. The body can habituate to diuretics and lose its ability of maintain a negative water balance. In other words, the body compensates for water loss by resisting water loss in the future. This is caused by hyperaldosteronism. Edema, as a result of water retention due to refeeding, is especially distressing. The client's awareness of swelling or edema may be imagined or the result of actual fluid retention. Medical risks due to diuretic use comes from the development of metabolic irregularities and exacerbating dehydration.

Again, metabolic risk may be minor unto itself with diuretic use but added to metabolic irregularities caused from vomiting, restricting and laxatives, risks may compound and escalate.

Withholding Insulin

Of all the many eating disorder behaviors, withholding inulin for those with insulin dependent diabetes mellitus (IDDM) is the most frightening single behavior I fear. I fear this over vomiting and severe restricting with associated weight loss. Withholding insulin is an effective way to lose weight and keep it off. This is due to the osmotic diuresis caused by high serum glucose levels that result in glucose being eliminated in urine. This successfully removes calories that would otherwise be used as energy and stored in the body. The problem is, it is easily lethal – virtually within minutes any time of any day. The chance of someone being found in a diabetic coma and medical professionals being available to intervene immediately is about zero.

Diabetic Coma

With not taking insulin as recommended, serum glucose levels increase to inordinately high levels so that those with IDDM can go into a coma. This could be lethal unless corrected immediately.

INADEQUATE GLUCOSE MONITORING

Aside from a deliberate attempt to induce a massive diuresis, a refusal to monitor glucose serum levels can be very dangerous. One will not know if serum glucose levels are normal, too high, or too low. The individual has no observable warning of critically high or low serum glucose levels. They will be flying blind with regard to diabetic status. This is a form of diabetic Russian roulette.

RANDOM INSULIN INJECTIONS WITHOUT MONITORING

As frightening as someone withholding insulin is, is someone not monitoring when they take insulin randomly. Taking an excessively high insulin dose for a given serum level, can result in an insulin induced coma. Between severe food restriction and alternating binge eating as well as on and off extreme exercise, serum glucose levels can wane to hopelessly unpredictable levels where guessing is not remotely reliable.

BRITTLE INSULIN DEPENDENT DIABETES MELLITUS

Complicating things further are those with brittle IDDM. These individuals have a difficult time stabilizing serum glucose levels even with close monitoring and appropriate insulin injections as it is. Poor monitoring and resistance to adhering to necessary insulin protocols can lead to precipitous end-organ damage. Irreversible blindness, kidney failure, as well as microvascular damage to other organ systems can develop.

Medical and Legal Consequences

From a legal perspective, anyone not controlling appropriate glucose levels should be considered incompetent to drive, fly an airplane, or operate heavy machinery. Also, the capacity to be able to care for children should be scrutinized.

For individuals who refuse to stabilize glucose levels and insist on driving, the police should be informed immediately to prevent a serious motor vehicle accident leading to injury or death. I remember a time when an 18 year old young woman who was going to leave my office, showing obvious signs of difficulty walking due to a lack of insulin use or glucose monitoring, refused to not drive home. She had a three hour drive after our visit. I called the police detachment and informed them of my concern. They said they would immediately stop her on the highway and take away her driver's license. I phoned her parents and urged them to take her to her doctor or emergency room for proper management of her diabetes.

Breastfeeding and Pregnancy

Breastfeeding typically eliminates 500 to 800 calories daily. It is hard to burn this many calories with even extreme exercise in a day. Sitting and expressing milk to eliminate this many calories must seem like a treat to some.

Pregnancy creates several sources of weight gain and is a serious body image threat to individuals when desperate measures to prevent weight gain and even lose weight can evolve. The mother and baby need to be monitored closely during pregnancy. Having said this, for some, the pregnancy state creates a kind of "time out" from the need to engage in eating disorder behaviors. This is more than just being good for the baby. Weight control urges, however, can return with a vengeance after delivery.

Self-Phlebotomy

Phlebotomy is the deliberate removal of blood from the venous system ordered by medical clinicians to determine the levels of various blood constituents such as electrolytes, minerals, blood proteins, calcium, blood cell determinants, and many more. This task is usually performed by lab technicians, nurses, and possibly medical doctors. Medical professionals are the most likely individuals to utilize self phlebotomy to cause weight loss because they are aware of its use, have the skills to carry it out as well have access to the equipment required.

Minor blood removal will not likely produce important medial problems aside from some dizziness but large amounts may cause syncope, anemia, and other blood value irregularities.

Rumination

Rumination is a behavior where individuals eat, then regurgitate stomach contents back into the mouth where food is chewed further and then swallowed again. This behavior may be repeated several times. It serves to allow the experience of eating and swallowing repeatedly without consuming more food to provide the same sensation.

Binge Eating and Related Behaviors

Binge eating is a common eating disorder behavior. With regard to eating disorder diagnostic criteria, binge eating has been clearly defined as stated below. There are other methods of eating large volumes of food in a day, yet not properly defined as binge eating. These include grazing or snacking throughout the day but not consuming large amounts of food in any given period of time. Individuals may say that they are in control of their eating as well. By the end of the day, however, an enormous quantity of food may have been eaten rivaling binge eating total daily caloric intake. At some level, how someone overeats becomes a moot point.

Binge Eating

Binge eating is recurring episodes of greater food intake than necessary in an abbreviated time frame and with an accompanying lack of self-control. Episodes of binge eating may last for several hours or may occur multiple times during the day. Definitions for eating disorder classifications change over the years so it is not critical that we stick to hard classification criteria. With regard to "greater food intake than necessary," this definition does not take into account celebratory eating such as for religious holidays, Friday nights at a university dormitory and so forth. Some with an eating disorder who say they binge and do consume inordinate quantities of food during these sessions, will say they feel in control of their eating. It is a choice and not the result of an uncontrollable urge to over indulge. They have carefully planned binges and chose to binge at will for any number of reasons. Regardless of semantics, ask individuals if they binge eat and agree on what is deemed a binge to them. If a client does not believe they binge eat but you as a clinician feel they do, work with that.

What Foods Do Those Who Binge Eat Actually Eat?

The answer is often any food available. Those with eating disorders, however, typically have preferred food choices. Food choices may be made based on taste and texture, ease of eating large quantities of food and ease for which food may be vomited. Some binge foods will be based on ethnic preferences. Binge foods are sometimes selected that individuals have been deliberately restricting for some time. Fats and carbohydrates are examples. Binge foods will often be sweet or salty such as what is felt to be "junk food" – ice cream, potato chips, baking, candy, and others. Those who binge on restaurant foods will only have food choices available from the menu.

When a client would say, with pride, they have not eaten chocolate for a year, I wouldn't have the heart to tell them they are likely doomed to experience a tsunami of chocolate binges down the road. It is very disheartening for those who restrict specific *fear foods* to eventually give in to binging on them. It is soul crushing and can lead to severe anxiety, depression, and suicidal thoughts and actions. Though binge eating by itself may not be a particularly risky behavior, the emotional fallout from it can be. Watch declining moods closely.

Where Do Binges Occur?

Binges can take place pretty much anywhere. When individuals say they binge eat we often assume it is in their homes. However, binges may take place in any of several locations. People binge in their homes, at work or school, restaurants, while walking down the street and so forth. In their home, they can binge in the kitchen, bedroom, bathroom, basement, stairwells, in the back yard or garden.

Bingeing becomes dangerous while driving. As with cell phone use while driving, bingeing can be too distracting with regard to the physical dynamics of eating and mental preoccupation with having to binge as well as drive at the same time. Binge eating while intoxicated presents the possibility of choking and asphyxiation. Binge eating may happen in conjunction with binge drinking or bingeing on pills such as sedatives or illicit drugs.

Other Dangers With Binge Eating

Many of the dangers associated with binge eating really come from the behaviors chosen to rid the body of food binged on namely those used to induce vomiting.

Binge eating is a major trigger to vomit. Therefore, the more one binges, the more one may be driven to vomit. When someone describes what a binge is for them, focus closely on how they deal with excessive food in their stomach.

Grazing

Grazing is a loose term to describe eating relatively small quantities of food over an extended period of time. Full-on binge-like quantities of food may be consumed in a day. Meticulously ask what someone means by grazing and estimate total daily quantities of food taken in and what they may do to rid the body of this food. Those who graze can easily vomit just as much as those who binge. Risks from the use of emetics, laxatives, or diuretics are still possible.

Grazing can occur in plain site of others without bringing attention to overeating. Some will "snack" all day at work without others noticing. Visits to the restroom will not be suspected by coworkers as opportunities to vomit. The same can happen at school, studying in a public library, in the home as well as walking or hiking for recreation. Grazing and exercising are two sets of eating disorder behaviors that can happen in full view by others without bringing awareness to one's self.

Trap-lines

Trap-lines, as in the context of eating disorders, refer to individuals purchasing food for binge purposes from a number of locations, one after the other. There are two kinds of binge trap-lines — *restaurant* and *grocery store* trap-lines.

A restaurant trap-line is when an individual will go to one restaurant, order food to eat in and then go to another restaurant and do the same. This can be repeated for many restaurants. Some will likely vomit in each restaurant toilets although, others may not vomit till arriving home or at another destination. Some may vomit into bushes, gardens, garbage cans in parks or along streets between restaurant visits. Others may vomit into bags or plastic food container, putting these into their purse or backpack to be disposed of at a later time.

Those who do not choose to attend a restaurant in person may order-in food from various restaurants in the same day without having to travel or fear they will be suspected of binge eating. It is more likely that, if ordering food to be delivered to their home, they have a place to vomit at will as long as others are not home.

Grocery store trap-lines are when individuals shop for binge foods in one grocery store then another, one after the other. The reason for this is so the one doing the shopping does not feel that cashiers will think they are purchasing food for binge purposes. Those with eating disorders often feel very exposed or obvious as someone who has bulimia. They think that "people must know" or that they stand out as someone who is bulimic. Another reason could be that different grocery stores have particular desired binge foods others do not.

Subjective Binges

Subjective binges are what those with bulimia believe to be a real binge but in reality are "normal" or small amounts of food eaten. Nutrition education should be provided explaining the difference between normal and small food quantities versus a real binge. The false belief one is bingeing will lead to the same efforts to deal with this through other compensating behaviors such as vomiting, laxative, and diuretic use as well as excessive exercise and restricting. Subjective binges create the same self-loathing and hopelessness as real binges.

Hoarding

Some will hoard food in their homes, car, college dorms, and other places. Hoarding provides an easily available food source to be accessed at will. No one needs to shop at the moment when fully stocked. Some hoard but do not consume the food but will instead let hoarded food rot before disposing of it or will throw it out before the "best before" date. It's as if individuals like to have food close by but because it may be deemed "forbidden" food, is not allowed to be consumed. This can be a very expensive process.

Stealing

Food can be very expensive especially if people purchase it in binge quantities. Some will not have ready access to funds. The options to acquire food are to, either steal food from grocery stores, order food in restaurants then leave before paying or steal money from family, partners, and friends. Some will steal wallets and purses from strangers.

Stealing creates important problems. If someone is caught stealing food from a grocery store, they will be prosecuted. They will then need a lawyer, which is very expensive, stand before a judge, and have to pay some form of restitution. A criminal record may be the result. A criminal record may exclude individuals from ever being able to be employed for a government position, non-profit society, education institute, or a job as a caregiver for vulnerable individuals such as children or those who are ill.

Those who steal food or money in order to purchase binge food may also have a history of stealing other items. They may steal for the thrill of it or because they desire something. They may be destitutes. Consider that someone could be a kleptomaniac and, if so, find resources to help them deal with this. Ask all clients if they have ever been legally charged or convicted of stealing food or any other items.

Dumpster Diving

Dumpster diving is the act of individuals climbing into dumpsters belonging to grocery stores with the purpose of acquiring free binge food. Some with eating disorders will do this as well as others who do not have an eating disorder. The amount of food thrown away from major grocery stores is staggering. Literally thousands of dollars worth of food daily is put into dumpsters. Whole hams, baking goods, and other foods are discharged without the wrapping being broken.

Risks may develop here due to the poor hygiene of dumpsters. As well, personal safety becomes an issue with being about in dark, shady parts of town at night. Should injury occur within a dumpster due to falling or choking on food, there may not be help close by anytime soon.

Catered Events

Catered events can be a significant and reliable source of binge food. Some individuals will deliberately seek employment in hotels or catering businesses. With being responsible for laying out food for smorgasbords and then cleaning up after meal events, there is often an ocean of food left over. This food then can be binged on during cleanup or may be removed to be eaten later. University students may look on-line to find out where there will be catered events on campus such as department lunches or dinners. They determine the time the event begins and plan to arrive just in time to binge on left over food or remove it to eat elsewhere.

Calorie Burning and Metabolism Altering Behaviors

There are several ways people believe they can burn calories. Altering metabolism artificially is one set of methods used.

Exercise

Exercise for the purpose of controlling weight and body image is a common practice for those with eating disorders. It is also a common practice for many others in society who do not have an eating disorder but who also wish to control weight and body image.

When enquiring regarding exercise practices we need to know the *kinds* of exercise chosen, *why* they have been chosen, *where* they are being carried out, the *intensity* with which they are being performed and the *endpoint* for their use.

Why Is Exercise Used?

Exercises serve several functions for controlling body image and weight.

- Burning calories
- Increasing metabolism
- Helping to decrease and control hunger
- Mentally occupying someone from focusing on food, eating and weight
- Physically occupying someone from the act of eating

Exercises, unto themselves, do not present critical risks generally. But their accumulative effects may add to risks associated with other eating disorder behaviors. They may also add risk to non-eating disorder sources of risk such as diabetes or congenital heart disease.

As an example, someone who is 5'5", 68 lbs (BMI = 11.3) and his eating disorder behaviors include:

- Restricting food intake to 500 calories daily
- Vomiting 3 sessions daily while vomiting 4–5 times per session, therefore, resulting in vomiting 12 to 15 individual times daily
- Using salt solutions as an emetic
- Taking 30 laxative tablets daily

He also has serious medical risks such as:

- Metabolic alkalosis with a potassium level of 1.8 mmol/L and serum magnesium of .66 mmol/L
- Dysrhythmias including runs of ventricular tachycardia and torsades de pointes
- Symptoms of syncope and palpitations

An exercise regime of running for two hours, using a rowing machine, stationary bicycle and weights for three hours in a gym with the intent of burning 600 calories daily can escalate serious medical risks contributing further to his near lethal metabolic state and dysrhythmias. Syncope while driving a car could injure or even result in killing himself or others. Here, exercise could push the individual into a lethal state when added to the other sources of risk. Assessing exercise use and resulting physical consequences is imperative.

Excessive exercise can contribute to the following serious health risks.

- Escalation of serious dysrhythmias
- Escalation of metabolic irregularities
- Sudden cardiac death
- Death from running into traffic

Less serious but significant health risks:

- Bone fractures especially in those with osteoporosis
- Chronic joint, spinous process, tendon and muscle pain
- Sprains of the ankles and knees
- Planter fasciitis

Clinicians need to accurately determine the kinds of exercises and, as important, the total daily energy expenditure. The total daily, weekly or monthly energy expenditure from exercise can be significant.

Injuries

Injuries for those with major exercise compulsions can lead to extremes of panic in response. The idea of not being able to exercise fully becomes intolerable. In my experience, those with exercise compulsion that cannot continue their extremes of exercise due to injury often resort to the most brutal engagements of other eating disorder behaviors in order to attain weight loss or prevent weight gain. For those who are dedicated exercisers and who have not had obvious body image or weight control issues prior to an injury, they may develop weight control drives after due to fear of gaining weight. It's almost as if there may have been a subconscious body image control drive lurking under the body awareness radar only to be released because of an injury. In particular, runners may be especially vulnerable.

Emotional risks that come with injuries can be:

- Panic and compulsions to escalate other eating disorder behaviors already in play
- Panic and compulsions to engage in other eating disorder behaviors never used before that could become dangerous such as vomiting or emetic, laxative and diuretic use as well as severe food restricting
- Panic leading to suicidal ideation and attempts as well as drug and alcohol use.

Other Exercise Interfering Causes

While injuries create a significant and usually temporary cessation of exercise, there are other factors that can do the same.

Illness such as the flu, infectious mononucleosis, COVID-19, inflammatory bowel disease, asthma, cardiac dysfunction as well as others can result in an athlete or compulsive exerciser to cease physical activities. For those who use a gym, a lack of funds can prevent exercise. A move to a different city, a change in job or attending a university may interfere with previously established physical activity regimes. Traveling with family on family trips can greatly interfere with routine exercise. Anxiety, depression as well as psychosis can interfere with someone's will to engage in exercise. Personal tragedy such as death of a loved one, ending of a relationship, job loss as well as other tragedies may contribute to a dark mood state.

Assessing Exercise Use

Different forms of exercise can present various capacities to control weight as well as risk. Aside from the *kinds* of exercise used, we need to know the *intensity* of a given exercise and make an estimate as to the total impact of all the kinds of exercises in play. This has been briefly touched on earlier.

For each kind of exercise we need to try to *quantify* its use. We can attempt to do this by determining the *number of times* an exercise is repeated (lifting weights, pushups, sit-ups, steps), *how long* or the *time* someone uses a particular exercise and possibly *how far* someone may travel (bicycling, walking, running, rowing).

We also need to know the *force* or *effort* required for a given exercise. As an example, we need to know how much weight someone is lifting or resistance to a rowing machine. Just knowing repetitions is not enough to assess total intensity for an exercise.

Ask as to how many calories someone wishes to burn during each exercise and total daily calorie count for all exercises in a day. Some may not be particularly focused on repetitions or length of time but the calorie count is deemed the most important goal of exercising.

Weight loss may not be the primary target for exercise. Some may want to shape their body, either to be trimmer or more athletic looking, regardless of weight obtained. Some want to increase the percentage of lean body mass, again, with weight control not being the goal. Less percent body fat is the goal. Others may engage in extreme exercise due to being elite athletes and are aiming to become Olympic athletes. Others just enjoy exercise for body and mind wellbeing.

In short, individuals may exercise for the following reasons:

- To control body image and weight
- They have an eating disorder
- To boost metabolism
- They enjoy exercise
- They are competitive athletes
- Exercise is a compulsion
- Exercise is a mechanism for socializing with family, friends, other athletes
- Exercise is part of therapy for recovery from drugs or alcohol abuse as well as depression and anxiety.

Metabolism Boosters

Aside from exercise, there are chemical methods used to increase metabolism. Some work and some don't but are still believed by some to do so.

Some chemical methods used for the intent of increasing metabolism are:

- Cigarette smoking
- Cocaine and some other illicit drug use
- Energy drinks
- "Diet pills"

Some *medical risks* due to using chemical metabolism boosters are:

- Stimulation of the heart to trigger tachycardia and lethal dysrhythmias
- Addiction
- Adding to further weight loss

Heating Blankets

Increasing body heat can increase the rate at which calories are burned. Working outside in the hot sun or inside a steel factory where molten steel is being poured will increase metabolic activity.

At home, wrapping one's self in an electric heating blanket as well as covering up in several layers of other blankets will increase body metabolism. It will also increase perspiration that will also cause further weight loss. Exercising under these blankets will further increase metabolism. Note that these activities can go completely unnoticed during night time sleeping hours.

Nonchemical Methods of Altering Metabolism

There are many nonpharmaceutical methods utilized to lose weight with little or no proof they work. These are a few options some choose.

- Taking vitamins B6 and 12.
- Eat before 7 p.m. as metabolism drops at night.
- Consuming apple cider vinegar, spices including black pepper, chili, and garlic, sea weed as well as green tea, cayenne pepper, and citrus water.
- Eating four 100 calorie meals will burn more calories than one 400 calorie meal.
- Eating high calorie foods earlier in the day.
- Any exercise
- Maintaining erect body posture, which involves the active use of several muscles, burns calories
- Consuming protein increases metabolism

- As with maintaining good posture, eating while standing
- Changing exercise patterns and nutrition will help to increase metabolism
- Binge after you eat a normal meal, as your metabolism will be up
- Eating cold foods and drinks
- Exercising in cold or hot environments

Negative calorie foods

Some foods are believed to burn calories while being digested. Some are believed to actually burn more calories than they provide the body.

Body Gauging Behaviors

For someone to want to lose weight, they must have some impression of their body size and shape. Assessment of body size and shape may be estimated, in part, through empirical methods as well as visual and tactile input. Regardless of empirical and sensory cues to form an assessment of body image, the imagination serves to have the most important input in this process.

Regardless of empirical or visual and tactile input, the mind can totally misread objective evidence of body size and shape. Someone with anorexia nervosa who is 5'4" who observes a weight on a floor scale of 85 lbs can still feel she weighs 400 lbs. If a mirror accurately reflects an emaciated, concentration camp like habitus, the individual can still see in her mind's eye a morbidly obese individual. As clinicians, we cannot depend on objective empirical or sensory data to sway individuals in accepting the realities of their health state.

Body gauging methods will not be dangerous unto themselves, but their impact on the drive to control body image and weight can be brutal. They serve as an unrelenting taskmaster that must be obeyed even if it results in death. Body gauging must be taken very seriously. We need to know the methods being used and the intensity of the grip they hold. It's as if the body gauging methods are holding a gun to the heads of those with eating disorders. It is important to know the target weight or physical symptom goals.

While using a scale is the only accurate and practical way to determine ones weight, the use of a mirror, tight clothing, measuring tape and other body gauging methods may be used to mentally assess weight. As an example, when someone can fit into a size 2 dress they may assume they weigh so much. When individuals say they know their weight, ask regarding how they determine this and is it likely to be quite accurate or just a wishful or punitive guess. Someone who sizes themselves using a clothing size, belt size or measuring tape may have previously determined their weight on a scale at the same time. Therefore, there may be some degree of accuracy.

The following are a few methods some use to assess body size, shape, and weight.

Scales

Scales used to weigh people are ubiquitous in society. They are in homes, work places, medical offices, gyms, health spas, as well as family and friends homes. For those who depend on these scales to determine an empirical value for their weight, they have a good selection to choose from.

Usually, individuals will choose one particular scale to weigh themselves regardless of there being access to others. The reasons for this may be that one scale is available most often and it is the one already calibrated as desired and not likely to be recalibrated between weighing sessions. The gym scale may read differently from the one in a medical office, home or at a friend's home. Any variation in how any given scale measures when compared to others is often not tolerable. Some will deliberately chose a scale that reads lower than others.

The most accurate lowest daily weight reading is usually felt to be first thing after one wakes up and after voiding. Little or no clothing is worn during a weigh-in. All other weight readings later in a day will typically be compared to this one.

Individuals may weigh themselves:

- First thing in the morning after waking and voiding
- Anytime during the day from none to dozens of times
- Weighing may happen after someone has just eaten and then after they have vomited or exercised to determine weight after food has been expelled or calories burnt off
- After a bowel movement or voiding
- After periods of restricting food and fluids
- To assess the weight of food consumed
- When first discovering one is pregnant, throughout pregnancy, immediately after delivery and weeks later after the pregnancy hormonal state has shifted to a non-pregnant state. This is when the fluid that had been retained during pregnancy will have been eliminated
- When qualifying for a weight determined sport such as rowing or wrestling as well as to keep their position on the team
- Due to pressure from an athletic coach to lose weight so they "look good" for the media
- To have the competitive psychological edge over other athletes such as show horse riders and curlers

Mirrors

As with the scale, the use of the mirror for gauging body size or shape can be an equally vicious taskmaster, and for some, may be more so.

Similarly, mirrors are ubiquitous. Unlike scales where there will usually only be one in a household, if at all, mirrors seem to occupy several rooms in homes. This includes every bathroom, most bedrooms, hallways and possibly in living rooms. Mirrors are located in purses, cars, gyms, spas, clothing, and other stores, education institutes and the work place. Reflective surfaces such as windows on stores serve to give individuals feedback as to how they look at a glance while walking down the street.

Although the visual image one sees in a mirror may be accurate to the visual cortex, the mind of those who are judgmental of their body size and shape can greatly exaggerate their interpretation of these images, typically in a negative context.

The mirror is used to scrutinize more than just total body shape or size, it can be used to nitpick given parts of the body. These could be the nose, thighs, knees, face, abdomen, love handles, arm fat and on and on. Regardless, the mirror typically focuses attention on the most disliked parts of the body. Focuses of body dissatisfaction can change. Some, at times, may like what they see in the mirror especially if body weight and size altering methods have been successful.

Clothing

Clothing is used to gauge body size or shape. While a weight on a scale or an image in a mirror or photograph provide body image data, clothing can provide powerful perceived body assessing information. There are several clothing body assessing methods.

Tight Clothes

Various pieces of clothing can be used as a body-gauging device. Tight trousers, especially jeans, leggings, and tops are used. Usually individuals choose a single piece of clothing to which they depend on as an assessing tool. If the piece of clothing fits snuggly then this is a signal to have to lose weight still. If it fits loosely then they have arrived at a body shape or size they have been aiming for.

Clothing Sizes

Akin to the use of tight clothes is the focus on clothing size. Some choose a clothing size for which they will feel comfortable in if they fit easily. Any sense of tight fitting clothes triggers the need to lose yet more weight. Clothing sizes as minimal as 00 is the goal for some. Some adults with anorexia nervosa will shop for children's clothing sizes.

Belt Size

Selecting a belt size to gauge body size can work similarly to tight clothes or clothing sizes. While one may achieve their goal of a small enough clothing or belt size the good feeling they get from this may not last. They then may wish to set an even smaller clothing or belt size in order to experience the same temporary euphoria.

Measuring Tape

A measuring tape can be used to measure several parts of the body, not just the waist. It can be used to assess the girth of the abdomen, hips, chest, upper arms and thighs. These are parts of the body for which individuals are usually the most dissatisfied with.

Photographs

Photographs have to be the upfront body assessing tool these days. Just a few decades ago photographs were taken with probably the only camera in a household. It also had to be used by someone with the skill to operate it. The exposed film had to be taken to a camera shop where there was the equipment to develop film and print copies onto photographic paper. Exposed slide or transparency film often had to be sent away to a large center for processing and this could take over a week for the developed slides to return. The cost of film as well as processing and printing was very expensive. Today, pretty much everyone has a high-resolution camera in their cellular phones. Perfect focusing, near perfect exposures and composition are essentially all immediate. And best of all, there is no cost to capturing excellent images. Some with eating disorders take thousands of photographs of themselves – selfies – as well as others.

These photos serve as an immediate record of how one looks now and the cell phone is a repository for past images that may go back several years. Photos automatically transfer to a new phone allowing a decade or more of photos to accumulate.

Another source of photographs may be from the family album that can be a cadre of older photos when individuals were in their young teens or even preadolescence.

Some with eating disorders will covet their body shape and size from earlier years. Older photos supply a benchmark or gold standard for current body image desires.

Aside from selfies and family photos, there is an ocean of photographs of other people on the internet. Photographs of emaciated individuals, whether models or other celebrities as well as the general public are accessible at will. Photos of morbidly obese people are also available, often associated with derogatory comments. These photos of emaciated and morbidly obese individuals are referred to as *thinspirational photos* downloaded from *pro-ana* and *pro-mia* websites.

Grabbing Body Parts

Some assess their body by grabbing different areas such as the wrists, thighs, arms, buttocks, hips, or abdominal fat.

Body Calipers

Body calipers, usually a device used by professionals to determine body fat percentage, may be used as well. There are instruments accessible to the public that allegedly electronically assess body fat.

Surgery and Other Cosmetic Altering Methods

In the eating disorder world, surgery serves many needs. There are many cosmetic surgery options to control weight, body shape, and size, remove unwanted skin lesions as well as to accent attractiveness including beauty.

Body Shaping as Well as Weight Reducing Surgery

Most surgery used to reduce weight also affects body shape. There are several surgical procedures at ones disposal. Some are very costly while others are not.

Breast Reduction

Although breast reduction is used to primarily reduce breast size for cosmetic or reconstructive purposes as well as to eliminate neck and back pain, it also removes fat tissue that has weight. Some will have a breast reduction exclusively to lose weight. For body shaping purposes, it may provide a more pleasing breast shape but also create more of an androgynous look or decreased sexual presentation. Plastic surgeons need be alerted to breast surgery for the purpose of weight loss. This must be deemed an unnecessary and extreme form of weight loss that only further buys into the destructive nature of ones eating disorder. For those where body shape is paramount, breast augmentation may be an option.

Liposuction

Liposuction is performed on the abdomen, thighs, hips, buttocks, neck, face, knees, and possibly elsewhere. It removes unwanted fat tissue, primarily for body shaping but also to lose weight.

Non-Weight Loss Cosmetic Surgical Procedures

Some cosmetic surgical procedures have no discernable weight loss capacity but are still used by those with eating disorders to deal with non-weight sources of body discontent. These can be a rhinoplasty, labiaplasty as well as liposuction around the knees and anywhere on the face and neck. Facelifts must be included here. Surgical removal of moles, trauma induced dermal scars or surgical scars, lipomas and other dermal tumors such as those associated with neurofibromatosis can be requested.

Risks Associated With Cosmetic Plastic Surgery

Plastic surgery can be very *expensive* and some individuals will spend tens of thousands of dollars on various surgical procedures for weight or body sculpting reasons. The Barbie Doll has been used as an ideal body shape for which individuals wish to replicate with multiple surgical operations.

A serious risk to some is that they will not like the outcome of surgery. Some operations are botched where the end result is terrible. Dissatisfaction may come from just not getting what they had been hoping for. The emotional cost can be catastrophic. If someone was unhappy about their body before surgery, regretted surgery compounds discontent. The financial cost of a revision can equal or surpass that of the original operation. Unless surgery is absolutely necessary, I discourage all cosmetic surgical procedures. If they refuse my suggestion, I then ask them to at least wait for a month or so before booking.

CoolSculpting or Cryolipolysis

Cryolipolysis is a commercial cosmetic procedure where intense cold is applied to fatty tissue. This destroys fat tissue in hopes of reshaping the body to a more desirable one. It is a costly procedure that may not give the hoped results.

Makeup

Applying makeup has been a mainstay for altering how someone looks for a few millennia. While diets, exercising, surgery and other weight and body image altering behaviors are at the beck and call of those with eating disorders, the use of makeup is also a factor. Makeup is used as an adjunct to other eating disorder behaviors but may also be used for other cosmetically altering purposes as the rest of the population would use it for.

Makeup can be applied in an attempt to further contribute to the *thin* or even emaciated look. Makeup can assist in making the face or knees appear thinner than they actually are. For other cosmetic reasons, makeup can be applied to hide blemishes including scars, nevuses, moles, capillary hemangiomas as well as others. As those with eating disorders can have an extreme loathing for unwanted weight, they also can develop a pathological dislike for non-weight related body dissatisfactions.

Gastric Bypass Surgery

The above surgical procedures result in weight loss and body shaping. Gastric bypass surgery serves only to create a way of losing weight with the intension of keeping weight off. Weight loss results due to a significant piece of nutrition absorbing bowel being removed. The total nutrition absorbing capacity of the bowel is reduced.

Medical consequences can be malabsorption syndrome, chronic diarrhea, adhesions and chronic abdominal pain. A large abdominal scar will remain. Weight loss expectations may not be deemed adequate leading to dissatisfaction with the outcome and further body loathing. It becomes yet another disappointment in an individual who has likely had years of life disappointments.

Restricting Eating Behaviors

Restricting food is a primary mechanism for losing weight, both for those with eating disorders and many who do not. *Dieting* has become a colloquial term used to describe restricting that presents in many forms often in fads. The medical definition of diet is where a set of recommended food choices, possibly in conjunction with exercise and other healthy life style options, have been determined for a particular health issue. These health concerns may be diabetes, hypercholesterolemia, gluten intolerance, hypertension, renal failure as well as several others. Weight loss may not be a goal. Sometimes a calorie increase is suggested.

Restricting food to decrease weight or stop weight gain is the restriction of calories. Calories, or kilocalories, is a measure to food *energy* intake. The determination of an individual's biological weight is amazingly complicated and rather poorly understood. Yet, a generally adopted belief in our society, including by some in the healthcare community, is that eating less leads to weight loss and eating more causes weight gain. At some level this is true, in part, but the factors that ultimately determine weight changes are many. Food *fasting* and *cleanses* are thought of as kinds of diets.

Factors That Affect Weight

There are many factors that affect weight. Some are eating disorder related while most are not.

- Genetics: height, weight, shape, gender, lean body mass, metabolism
- Kinds of food

- Quantities of food consumed
- Metabolic status
- Energy expenditure
- Some medications
- Fluid shifts
- Hormonal changes
- Urination and bowel movements
- Age
- Gender
- Race
- Cultural body size and shape preferences – the unnaturally thin body coveted in developed countries versus the voluptuous body of a woman from Trinidad
- Ethnic food choices as well as the physical activity of different cultures (playing video games all day verses skiing or diving for pearls)
- Breastfeeding
- Pregnancy, delivery and post-pregnancy period
- Surgical removal of body tissue or additions to a body such as breast implants
- Water loss through perspiration and respiration
- A multitude of eating disorder behaviors
- Intravenous fluids
- Percent lean body mass
- Set-point weight
- Illness
- Ambient temperature
- Core body temperature
- Shivering
- Blood loss
- Malignant or benign tumors

Although decreasing food or calorie intake sounds simple – "just eat less" – there are several dozens of methods or behaviors those with eating disorders may utilize to meet this goal. Understanding what these behaviors are providing clinicians is an understanding of the mindset of those with eating disorders. They teach us about the degree of desperation and resulting creative thought processes that grip those with eating disorders. It also teaches us about the etiologies of evolving medical and psychological risks.

Calorie Assessing Behaviors

There are three methods of assessing food quantities to assure one has not eaten too much. One is empirical through using precise mechanical measuring devices. The second is approximating with the use of scientifically derived food data guides. The third is full-on guessing.

Measuring Food Volume

One empirical method of determining food quantity and, therefore, calorie content is by measuring food with *utensils calibrated for volume* such as measuring spoons or measuring cups. They provide quite an accurate, predictable and controllable measurement of foods, both solid and liquid. Food volume can be determined as well by using a food weighing scale. Some food containers have labels that provide some degree of accuracy of volume determination and therefore food weight and calorie determination.

Weighing Food

Food weigh scales provide a precise measurement by weight of food products for both solids and liquids. As with volume measurements of food, calorie content can be fairly accurately predicted. Certainly, more than by guessing.

Weighing food is sometimes attempted by using a floor scale. That is, individuals will measure their body weight first, then eat, after which they weigh themselves again to determine the weight of food consumed. From this, they can guess with regard to the caloric content of food taken in.

Reading Labels on Food Containers

Labels on food wrapping or cardboard and plastic food containers may provide data regarding:

- Food weight
- Food volume
- Nutrient content such as protein, carbohydrate, and fat.
- Minerals including sodium
- Vitamin content
- Calorie content per serving
- Soda, sport, and power drinks may provide information regarding what is listed above and also caffeine and electrolyte content. Carbohydrate data may be specifically identified, in part, by sugar content

Calorie Counting

Calorie counting is a near ubiquitous eating disorder behavior. Determining the true calorie content of consumed food may be quite accurate or a guestimate. Calorie counting is a method of attempting to put a firm limit on calories consumed when eating snacks or meals as well as determining the total daily calorie intake.

Individuals attempt calorie counting certainly by reading food labels, assessing servings and mechanical measuring methods. Although counting calories is important to many, some do not factor in calories when weighing, measuring or determining the number of servings available. There may be health or fitness purposes to food management.

Counting Servings

Counting servings is another approximate way of determining food energy input. As with weight and volume determinations, servings can be converted to calorie content.

Serving determinations for various foods have been defined by nutrition scientists. Medical food guides provide what has been accepted as food servings through size, weight or volume determination. Some values are very precisely stated such as "a serving of rice is half a cup." Others are quite loose such as "a medium sized apple is one serving." These formal food guides are really designed for the general public in an attempt for them to estimate what kinds of foods are recommended and the number of servings suggested. They are poor at making appropriate food recommendations based of ethnicity, gender, age or energy expenditure. Food guidelines for those with health considerations such as diabetes, pregnancy, gluten sensitivity, malabsorption syndrome, inflammatory bowel syndromes as well as several others will be better defined than those for general public use.

Guessing

Regardless of the empirical means of determining calorie value of food, guessing will be likely an option for many. Some guesses will be close while others may be way off.

When enquiring regarding an individual's food and especially calorie intake have them describe as precisely as they can how they determine calorie values. Although many are well versed in calorie determination, others are very poor at it. There are so many myths as well as outright disinformation regarding food energy assessment that clinicians need to be very sure of the accuracy of the information they collect. Why is this? Clients sometimes overestimate the calorie worth of some nutrients. Other times they may underestimate. Clients may be eating far less calories than we assess from their distorted history. If we estimate that a daily food intake is 1200 calories, based on the client's account of what they eat but in reality are taking in only 400 calories daily, we can greatly underestimate their medical risks. We tend to think of many with eating disorder as experts in nutrition, as they themselves often believe they are, but this may be far from the truth for a given individual.

Calorie Reducing Behaviors

Although empirical calorie assessing methods exist, there are many other ways individuals attempt to limit food intake.

Skipping Meals and Snacks

One way to reduce food intake is to skip individual meals and snacks. Relatively large quantities of food can be deleted from a typical daily intake without vomiting.

Meal and Snack Reduction

Eating smaller snacks and meals will reduce intake to a degree. Some may skip meals and snacks at times and only reduce meal and snack quantities other times.

Reducing the Volume or Size of Food

Reducing the volume or size of certain foods cuts down on calories. Some foods such as fruit are described as small, medium, and large. Choosing a smaller piece of fruit will decrease calories. Drinking smaller quantities of liquids will also achieve the same. Volume reduction can be achieved for those who usually put a tablespoon of butter on mashed potatoes but instead put a teaspoon worth or none at all. If someone uses two tablespoons of sugar in their coffee, they may choose one tablespoon instead. A cup of sugar usually listed in a recipe for cookie doe may be deliberately reduced to half a cup.

Reducing the Weight of Food

As some will reduce the volume of food they eat, consuming less weight of food can achieve similar results. As an example, if a recipe for chili con carne ordinarily requires one pound of hamburger, half a pound may be tried instead. Weight determination can be made with a home food scale but also in grocery stores where fruits, vegetables, and bulk foods can be weighed.

Reducing the Percentage of Food

Where volume or weight reduction of food is important for some, many choose to think in terms of percentage food reduction. Some will say to themselves "I'm going to eat 25% less in a day" or "I'm going to cut carbs in half." Weight or volume assessments are used to calculate percentage food reduction. As an example, an individual might use half a pound of flour instead of one pound in order to cut calories by 50%. Another might reduce eating a pint of yogurt in one go to a half-pint in order to create a 50% reduction in calories.

Vegetarian Diets

Vegetarian diets have become very popular in the last few decades. This is due to increased awareness of health and environmental risks related to raising animals for food production and the effect consumption of meat has on health in humans as well. Concerns regarding animal cruelty have gained increasing attention too. Vegetarian diets have also become a staple in the weight loss diet world.

Those with eating disorders may have adopted vegetarian diets based on genuine health and humanitarian purposes. Vegetarian diets can, however, become an excuse to not eat high-energy foods from many sources such as dairy products including eggs and cheeses as well as meat.

Fad Diets

Fad diets have been around for decades if not hundreds of year. A fad diet is any diet that comes into the public consciousness as one that promises weight loss or health benefits that are usually too good to be true and often have no basis in science. Although weight loss can be impressive with some fad diets, their capacity to keep weight off will probably be a failure. If weight loss can actually be maintained, then the individual likely has developed an eating disorder utilizing restricting eating behaviors as well as calorie burning or purging methods.

When fad fat reducing diets became less popular, carbohydrates became the new vilified food. Some of these carbohydrate reducing diets would allow almost any quantities of unmeasured meat, which contain high percentages of protein and fat but lettuce had to be weighed. These diets became a huge success as more weight loss seemed to happen quicker than with other previous diets. The degree of weight loss was very impressive to be honest. Needless to say, these diets had the most profound rebound weight gain by the end of a year or so. Also, it was discovered that low carbohydrate, high protein diets could be fatal.

Keto diets seem to be the latest in diet trends. Some versions claim that a diet should consist of 75% fat, 10–30% protein and no more than 5% or 20 to 50 grams of carbohydrates daily. These diets, again, deprive the body of essential nutrients that can lead to health problems including heart disease. Weight loss is not sustainable and can result in adopting an eating disorder.

As an editor of an international journal of eating disorders, I remember reviewing a submitted article that professed a junk food diet. The theory being that if people ate their favorite snack foods as their meal, they would eat less regular food and not gain weight because they would not be craving for deserts and other sweet and salty foods after meal time. I deep-sixed the article. It just shows how diets keep popping up to yet again promise weight loss programs that in the end don't work and probably causes weight gain ultimately.

Safe Foods

Safe foods are foods that are deemed "safe to eat" from a calorie perspective. The assessment of what a safe food is, however, is quite unique for each individual. "Safe foods" are really in the mind of the beholder. While some feel that low fat and protein foods are not safe foods because they are high in calories, others chose them because they tend to satiate hunger for longer periods of time and help prevent overeating. A feeling of contentment or having eaten enough occurs with smaller quantities of high-energy foods.

Food in liquid form may be seen as either safe or not. Liquids tend to go down easier and are often tolerated better. Homemade shakes or commercial nutrition supplements can contain a broad variety of nutrients and may be considered a meal in themselves. Others consider liquid nutrition replacements fear foods because they are high in calories per volume. They are often disliked on taste alone. Some prefer to think of food as medicine.

Fear Foods

Fear foods are foods that are avoided because they are believed to especially cause weight gain. Typically fatty foods or snack foods are included. However, any food can be deemed a fear food. These are the opposite of safe foods essentially.

Medication Avoidance

As mentioned earlier, there are a number of medications that are avoided because the active ingredients are feared to cause weight gain. Also, the tablets or liquids they are prepared in themselves have calories even though minuscule. Individuals are able to determine the calorie content of some medications from surfing the internet. Some medications might have 5 to 10 calories per dose. Either the medication will not be taken because of fear of this negligible calorie amount or allowances will have to be made to reduce the equivalent calorie worth other ways. This could be accomplished with food restriction, increased exercise, vomiting or any number of other eating disorder behaviors.

Offering Food to Others

Offering food to others is a convenient way to reduce food that is expected to be eaten when eating with others. If someone with an eating disorder is expected to eat with others, they will feel trapped knowing they are expected to finish the food in front of them. Offering food to others such as deserts, French fries, or half a hamburger may work in some situations. This will be more likely successful when eating with people who are unaware of the eating disorder. Attempting this with family, a partner or friends who know of the eating disorder will be harder if not impossible.

For those eating in a restaurant, uneaten food can be packed up in a doggy bag. After leaving the restaurant, it may be given to someone on the street. This helps to get rid of the guilt associated with throwing away good food and it feels like a humanitarian act feeding someone who is hungry.

Ordering Sauces on the Side

For food that typically comes with sauces such as salad dressing, gravy, sweet and sour sauce, plum sauce and others, ordering sauces on the side can be left uneaten with others present who do not suspect this is a restricting ploy. As well, just declining that these be included with the meal at all is a way to decrease calorie intake. Sauces tend to have a high fat and sugar content so are seen to be high calorie sources as they usually are.

From a recovery perspective, high calorie foods containing fats or protein are advised for those with eating disorders as they are satiety foods that actually reduce hunger spikes which is good for those who binge eat. Foods with high sugar content will likely cause spikes in serum glucose resulting in insulin peaks that in turn lower serum glucose resulting in frequent hunger.

Some salad dressings have a calorie content of over 190 calories for a 2 tablespoon serving. Others have less. Vinaigrettes tend to have lower calories.

Another way of cutting caloric intake is by ordering lunch, child-sized or senior size meals. They also will be less expensive. To others, eating with someone with an eating disorder but who are unaware of the disorder, declining sauces and ordering smaller meals looks "healthy" or that the person is "in control" of their food.

Declining Side Orders Including Desserts

Akin to not eating sauces or ordering smaller size meals is declining side orders. If side-orders such as French fries, onion rings, poutine, salads, toast, bacon and so forth are declined, this can reduce the total calorie content of meals significantly. Declining desserts also reduces the total calories of a meal. This makes meals a bit less expensive as well. Some may not be thinking in terms of calorie reduction only but also fat, sugar and protein reduction.

Picking Apart Food

Some individuals pick food apart so they can scrutinize the food content in mixed foods. Sandwiches, wraps, hamburgers, salads, stews, Chinese food are a few examples. Some do this to secure the notion that they know what is going into their body for sure – a control behavior. There may be no attempt to remove food. Others may look for food they can extract because of intolerable calorie or nutrient content. Cheeses or meats especially may be removed. The bread from a sandwich that may have butter or mayonnaise spread on it may be removed while the remaining contents are eaten. Some will remove the bun from a hamburger only to eat the meat, lettuce and tomato. For those on a keto diet, hamburger buns can be replaced with lettuce. Some restaurants offer keto meals where lettuce or keto buns are on the menu.

Gum and Candy Calories

Chewing gum and sucking on candy can be strongly adopted or refused by those with eating disorders as an eating disorder behavior.

Those who chew gum or suck on candies will likely choose sugarless versions of them. They tend to be used as a distraction from eating by giving the mouth a sense of pleasure with having something to taste as well as something to chew on or suck on. In the short term, they may also curb hunger to some degree. It is also a reminder to not put anything else into the mouth. The thought of food getting mixed in with gum acts as a deterrent. Sugarless gum and candies are seen as a very low calorie way of restricting.

Others avoid chewing gum and sucking on candies as they all have at least a few calories, however minimal. The calorie value may only be 5–10 calories per stick of gum or piece of candy, but this is interpreted as adding to the total daily calorie intake. This is similar to those who refuse medications because of the miniscule calorie content of each tablet or teaspoon of liquid.

Though chewing a piece of gum sounds like a trivial eating disorder behavior, individuals have said they have lost 30 lbs doing this. Chewing gum by itself is not dangerous but the resulting weight loss can be. Never underestimate the importance of any behavior in aiding individuals reaching extremes of physical compromise.

Throwing Food Away

Throwing food away, so as not to be eaten, can be an easy task or very difficult one. Food may be chosen to be thrown away in many situations.

Reasons for throwing food away can be:

•   Food is not enjoyable

- Food contains unwanted calories
- An individual does not want to become fat
- An individual is not hungry
- Food is spoiled or rotten
- Food is past "best by" date
- The expectation to have to eat

The ease or difficulty with which someone has the opportunity to throw food away depends on whether there are convenient disposal bins or whether there are people around that would disapprove of throwing food away.

As mentioned regarding restaurant food, uneaten food can be left on a plate so others will throw it away or it can be packed up then thrown away in the restaurant restroom garbage bin as well as anywhere outside of the restaurant.

For those eating with family, a partner or others, getting rid of food can be difficult if not impossible. This is true for home meals or those in restaurants. Food can be taken unnoticed during a meal by putting it in a napkin to be disposed of later. Chewed food can be spit into a napkin and later disposed as well. If food can be removed from the plate unnoticed at home, it could be fed to the family dog at the dinner table.

Uneaten food may be disposed of in garbage containers, flushed down a toilet, given to pets, or temporarily stored in bags or plastic food containers to be thrown away at a later time. This same food can certainly be eaten later, if desired. A car is an excellent food storage space for food to be later eaten or disposed of.

Chewing and Spitting

Some chew and spit food in order to have the enjoyment of food aroma, flavor and texture. As well, they have the assurance that they have not consumed many calories yet having some semblance of having eaten.

Licking Chopsticks or a Fork

Similar to chewing and spitting, but likely providing a sense of consuming extremely low calories, licking eating utensils dipped in broth, soup, sauces, chili or stews suffices for some. It provides some food aroma and flavor but not any satisfaction from food texture.

Dark Plates

Some find eating off of a dark plate an asset as a dark surface psychologically is believed by some to encourage eating less.

Sugar Substitutes

There are sugar substitutes that promise very low calories or none at all. They are synthetic or natural. The hope of using these products is that calories typically found in sugar will not be consumed and this is true. The problem is sugar-free foods do not help to prevent the total daily intake of food. The body knows when it is being cheated and wants to replace the energy restricted. That is, the calories that are hoped to be eliminated from the diet by eating foods with sugar substitutes will likely be added somewhere else in the day.

Selective Eating

Some with eating disorders have very selective food choices. They may restrict certain food groups because of their high calorie content or carbohydrates because they are believed to be a major cause of obesity. Some may choose to eat only a few foods that may be somewhat filling in the moment as well as very low in calorie content, carrots and celery being examples.

Children can adopt selective eating habits or be seen to be "picky eaters". These behaviors are usually considered normal and often go away on their own. However, when selective eating persists in children, adolescents or adults and body image or weight control is not an issue, then a diagnosis of *avoidant/restrictive food intake disorder (ARFID)* needs to be considered. Those with ARFID should be observed closely as they may be at risk of developing anorexia nervosa or bulimia. A given individual can be diagnosed with ARFID as well as anorexia nervosa or bulimia. That is, someone may refuse to eat a particular food because they do not like the color of it, white food being and example, and at the same time refuse to eat white rice, potatoes or white bread because they are carbohydrates that they fear cause weight gain.

Fluid Restriction

While food restriction or purging the body of food are mainstays of restricting calorie behaviors, fluid restriction is common. Water and other fluids are quite heavy – 1 gallon of water = 8.35 lbs and one cubic foot of water weights 62.43 lbs. Therefore, small decreases in water intake or loses due to voiding can make a measurable difference in weight.

Water is not exclusively taken into the body through drinking, as many foods contain water. Restricting solid foods can be a cause of considerable dehydration without restricting fluids deliberately. Fruits and vegetables tend to have high water content. Dehydration can be caused deliberately but also inadvertently without an individual being aware this is happening through their eating disorder behaviors.

Eating Various Foods With Different Flavors

Eating foods with different flavors can heighten the enjoyment of eating without having to rely on eating more.

Delaying Eating

Delaying eating is a way of allowing hunger to pass. Sometimes hunger or cravings pass on their own. At times, they do not. Delaying eating can reduce impulsive drives to eat including binge eating. This is similar to delaying having a cigarette when trying to quit smoking.

Chewing Several Times

Chewing food several times before swallowing is a way of delaying food intake and is similar to chewing and spitting by providing prolonged taste and texture pleasure. The hope is that by delaying eating as a result of slow chewing, the individual will be able to resist consuming more. Those that do this are able to receive some food enjoyment, some hunger relief and, hopefully, consume less food overall. It does provide some nutrition that skipping meals does not.

Set Utensils Down Between Bites

A simple way to delay the total time a meal is completed is by putting eating utensils down between bites of food. Again, this can allow for binge urges and hunger to pass and some degree of satiety to set in with eating less.

Paint Nails or Whiten Teeth

Painting nails is really a distracting technique but certainly can delay eating. Painting nails is seen as a finicky process. The thought of messing up wet painted nails with food while eating is repulsive to some. Whitening teeth cannot be done while eating. It serves both as a distraction and delaying technique.

Chopsticks

Unless someone was raised in a family who used chopsticks from a very young age, the rest of us can only barely cope using them. Thus, using chopsticks will typically slow the eating process.

Eat With the Opposite Hand

Most eat with their dominant hand. Using the other hand will feel clumsy and likely take longer.

Hunger Reduction

Aside from delaying eating there are other methods for attempting reducing hunger. Reducing hunger may help to prevent unwanted eating as well as bingeing. Some can resist eating when very hungry but many may not. Successful hunger suppression is a key to not consuming unwanted calories.

Fluid Loading

As with solids, liquids can relieve hunger. Liquids without calories such as water are the most desired for hunger suppression.

Water is an ideal substance for filling up on. It's either free or very inexpensive. It is ubiquitous in society and is 100% calorie free. It can be consumed in the direct eyes of others without suspicion of it being used as an eating disorder behavior.

Fluid loading is often carried out just prior to being weighed by clinicians. Individuals may do this when going to be weighed on a hospital ward or in the doctor's or dietician's office.

Foods With Fiber

Fiber in the form of bran or psyllium are common products used to keep bowel movements regular and prevent constipation. They are also used for general dieting and for those with eating disorders. Cellulose cannot be digested in humans. Therefore, it passes through the bowel intact. Individuals consume fiber as it provides space occupying bulk in the stomach and intestines creating a sense of fullness as regular food would do but with lower calories.

Although pure fiber is sugar free, much sugar is often added to fiber products in order to provide a palatable taste. The calorie content of fiber on it's own is negligible but added sugar supplies a significant calorie content.

Peppermint to Decrease Hunger

Peppermint has a reputation for curbing hunger. It can be provided in candy form or teas.

Cigarettes

Cigarette smoking is used by those with eating disorders for several reasons. It can act as a distraction from eating as well as keeps the mouth and hands occupied. Nicotine also suppresses appetite and is believed, by some, to increase metabolism that, in turn, burns more calories. Cigarettes are very expensive and if funds are spent on purchasing cigarettes, then there may be no extra money for food. This serves as a financial incentive to restrict.

Cotton Ball Diet

Just as it sounds, some will eat cotton balls to act as a stomach distending substance that can curb hunger. Cotton does not digest therefore there is no risk of calorie absorption. Most "cotton balls" are made of polyethylene. They contain toxic substances that can be absorbed. Cotton balls can cause bezoars that may result in bowel obstruction.

Chemical Appetite Suppressants

Some have been in prescription form and others may be obtained over the counter in pharmacies. Others may be acquired through mail or courier services. Some will make bulk purchases of appetite suppressants, metabolism boosters or laxatives along with others who have an eating disorder in order to keep costs down.

Spoiling Food

Food can be spoiled through deliberate sabotage or made undesirable through mental imagery.

Put Strong-Tasting Substances on Food

Too much of any strong tasting substance will ruin the taste of food. Examples are pepper, mustard, garlic, salt, chili or curry spices, onion or garlic salt as well as hot peppers. These are readily available condiments many of which will already be in the spice cupboard of most homes. Horseradish and hot cayenne based sauces (Buffalo wings) are possible choices.

The taste of food can be spoiled with almost any substance aside from what has already been mentioned. Mounds of sugar and non-hot savory spices can be mixed in with food.

Other Substances That Can Ruin the Taste or Desire for Food

Aside from food based additives, non-food based substances will ruin food as well. These can include cleaning solutions such as dish or laundry soap and floor cleaners. Food spoilers can be toxic and possibly caustic resulting in mouth, throat and esophageal chemical burns. Liquids such as water, vinegar, pop as well as milk pored onto food can ruin the desire to eat due to a disgusting flavor or the liquefying of food.

Food Associations

Mental associations can be made with food. The vile image of one's self being a pig or cow, for example, can be deliberately conjured up before or while eating. Food, itself, can be mentally imaged as being a plate full of worms, maggots, rotten food or hair. These images can discourage one from eating.

Microwave Food Too Hot to Eat

Food can be microwaved hot enough to cause burns of the mouth and throat. This can be a deterrent to wanting to continue eating. It may also be a form of punishment for attempting to eat in the first place.

Motivating Behaviors

Those with eating disorders use various methods to motivate themselves to control weight.

Mantras

A mantra is a short saying that can be spoken out loud or in the mind. It is usually a positive thought that bolsters ones mood and esteem. For those with eating disorders it could be a saying that encourages eating disorder motivations. For some, it could be to aid with motivation for recovery.

Write Your Weight on One Hand and Goal Weight on the Other

Writing one's current weight on one hand and goal weight on the other will remind an individual of their current weight and the weight they ultimately want to be. When wanting to, they will immediately see these two figures as a reminder that if they eat they will not reach their goal, or indeed, could become fat.

Sleep Over Six Hours a Night Will Increase Metabolism

Some believe that sleeping over six hours and possibly longer will help to burn more calories. Another reason for sleeping longer is the longer one sleeps, there is less time in the day to think about food as well as eat or binge.

Find an Eating Disorder Buddy

Those with active eating disorder behaviors and are in the mindset to pursue extremes of weight loss often feed off of the encouragement of others with eating disorders. Where do those with active eating disorders meet?

They might meet one another at school on the basketball or swim team, amongst peers as well as in the work place. However, a major meeting place is in eating disorder programs. For those hospitalized or in residential programs they meet on the wards. They meet in hallways, at group meals, as well as nutrition, therapy and yoga groups. They sneak between their rooms when they hope staff will not notice. People can meet also in outpatient group settings. Once having met in program settings, many carry on their relationship after. They certainly can meet in the community in person but it is likely they connect on social media. Like-minded groups with eating disorders can meet on line and carry on supporting destructive eating disorder attitudes and behaviors. Because of the recidivism of those not wanting to recover, eating disorder buddies will reconnect when readmitted coincidently during the same treatment stay.

When one person is readmitted to an eating disorder program, a buddy or friend can support eating disorder behaviors from the outside. Accomplices may bring laxatives, diuretics, sedatives as well as alcohol and street drugs into the hospital or residential ward. Binge foods can also be smuggled in.

Buddies can share behaviors they themselves use to lose weight, toxic mantras and websites that support eating disorder motivations. Buddies can also meet in person then binge and vomit together.

On the other hand, individuals will align with others that want to recover. There are peer support groups. Trained peer support workers assist those wanting to recover similar to alcohol and narcotics recovery programs.

Eating in Front of the Mirror

Eating in front of a mirror brings an immediate awareness of how one looks while eating. For anyone, even those without an eating disorder, this will not be a pretty site. For some with eating disorders, the vision of seeing one's self eating would be intolerable. It would be a disgusting image.

Wear a Rubber Band

As some wear a rubber band on a wrist to snap when reaching for a cigarette in an attempt to quit smoking, the same may be done for those who want to interfere with urges to eat and binge.

Stack Magazines and Remove Them

Some will stack magazines that total their current weight. As they lose weight, they remove the equivalent of weight loss in magazines from the stack. Watching the stack decline in height brings further encouragement to lose weight.

Time Rules

Many with eating disorders have time guidelines or rules regarding eating, restricting, vomiting, exercising, or the use of other eating disorder behaviors. These may be loosely adhered to or become harsh taskmasters.

Eat By a Certain Time

This rule dictates that one can eat a designated meal, breakfast, lunch, dinner or snacks by a specific time. If they don't then they have to skip the meal but eat by a certain time later. The meal or snack is then deliberately skipped and, therefore, will not add to the daily calorie count.

Eat at a Certain Times

Here, the rule is to eat *at* a given time or "right on time." Eating before or after is forbidden. If this does not happen, then the meal is skipped. Eating cannot happen until the next designated meal or snack.

Eat During a Given Time Period

This rule dictates that food is to be eaten between two times. As an example, one might set a rule that breakfast be eaten between 8:00 and 8:20 am. If food is eaten before or after this time frame or not eaten at all, then the rule has been broken.

Consequences of Meeting or Not Meeting Time Rules

A broken time rule can create guilt and shame as well as a sense of failure. Also, there may need to be punishment for this failure and various options for reparations may be drawn upon. Self-harm, missing the next meal or binge eating may be considered.

Time Rules May Be Created in Conjunction With Non-Eating Disorder Objectives

While time rules can be triggered by eating disorder dictates, there may be other factors that contribute to this. *Obsessive-compulsive disorder* may be linked to food related time considerations.

Rules Aiding Restricting

Individuals can make up rules regarding any aspect of their eating disorder control focus. Some apply to restricting attitudes and behaviors.

Eat Nothing White

White foods are often associated with foods that cause excessive weight gain. These can be white bread, table sugar, ice cream, milk and fat on meats. Food itself does not have to be white, such as a lot of baking, but these will often be made with white flour, sugar and milk. Ice cream of any kind, including chocolate and Rocky Road, may be assumed to be made with white dairy products. Certainly anything made with lard or has mayonnaise in it is game for scrutiny.

Never Eat Out

For some, eating out means eating high calorie fried foods such as hamburgers and French fries. Restaurants may trigger binge eating. Eating out may mean going to a mall and eating in a food court where there will be several restaurants serving quickly prepared foods. Food courts not only provide a source of varied restaurants but restrooms where one can vomit and are easily accessible. Serial restaurant cruising in the same food court can go unnoticed.

A Glass of Water Every Hour

Some have a rule of drinking water every hour. This is to curb appetite on a regular basis. For those that have been restricting, hunger can be constant requiring frequent relief, if only temporary.

Weigh Yourself Twice a Day or More

This rule guarantees that there will be a built-in watchdog tool to catch weight shifts through the day. The observed weight on a scale can bring delight with evidence of weight loss or possibly no weight gain but may, instead, bring distress with viewing an unwanted number on a scale.

Stop Eating in Your Bedroom or Car

Some will have a habit of eating in particular designated binging places. This can be in the car, bedroom or other reliable sites. These become state dependent triggers to binge eat.

Only Eat in Front of Others

Eating in front of others can be a deterrent from someone overeating. This can be because family or friends who know about the eating disorder will be watching for untoward behaviors such as bingeing, restricting or going to the restroom to possibly purge. Eating with those who are unaware of an eating disorder, will still provide a social setting where overt overeating or restricting behaviors are kept in check.

Never Eat in Secret

For some, eating in secret is a trigger to binge eat, vomit, exercise or also to take laxatives or diuretics. Eating around others can provide some barrier to eating disorder behaviors.

Never Eat Out of Food Containers

Eating out of food containers can serve as a cue to overeat. These containers could be for ice cream, yogurt, Chinese food and other food choices. Potato chips, nacho chips and candies come prepackaged. For some, they are unable to stop eating till the whole package is finished. While some snack foods come in quantities meant for one person, many come in larger containers meant for use by several individuals or for one person to take limited portions from time to time.

Rituals

Some adopt faithfully regular and invariable behaviors that become a keystone to eating disorder adherence. Some of these rituals are as follows.

Cutting Food

Some cut food into a specific number of pieces or a particular size. The act of cutting can delay eating marginally. Small pieces of food can then be eaten one at a time. Single pieces can then be chewed multiple times, slowly thus possibly helping to reduce the total consumption for a meal. Utensils can be put down while one is chewing, further slowing the eating process. As mentioned earlier, cutting food, putting utensils down then chewing slowly all help to allow consumed food the time to curb appetite reducing the urge to eat what would be felt to be too much. Appetite reduction is the result of stomach distention, nutrient absorption and hormonal triggers.

Specific Cutlery

Some choose specific eating utensils. This may be because one has a particular liking for some cutlery. It also may be because it aids in slowing the eating process down. Some will choose to eat with doll cutlery, doll bowls and plates. Eating with such small cutlery will allow an individual to only eat in very small quantities.

One Particular Bowl, Plate, Glass or Cup

A small plate or bowl puts a limit on the total area food can be presented to eat from. Small drinking glasses and cups define distinct limits of liquids.

Eating Clockwise or Counterclockwise

Some choose to eat either clockwise or counterclockwise on a plate full of food. This could be related to obsessive compulsive traits or a superstitious gesture.

Not Allowing One Food To Touch Each Other

Some will refuse to eat if one food touches another. There may be a sense of spreading "contamination" from one food to another. This will not be due to fear of bacterial contamination but of calorie transfer from one food to another.

Food is Eaten in a Specific Order

Some will want to eat food in a particular order. That is, to eat one food before the other. Some will eat the least calorie rich food first and then move onto other foods with more calories. As an example, a person would eat the salad first, because it has the least calories per weight, then move onto vegetables that have higher calories and finally rich foods such as cheese or meat. The idea here is an attempt to fill up on lower calorie foods first with the possibility of not wanting to eat the richer food as hunger resides.

Superstitious or Religious Meaning

Food rituals can take on superstitious or even religious context. This is akin to "Step on a crack, you'll break your mothers back." That is, something bad will happen if one doesn't adhere to the rules. Food rituals may not have anything to do with weight control. Or, they may serve to meet the dictates of superstitious needs as well as body image control ones.

Not Eat Mixed Foods

Some will not eat mixed foods such as stews, chili con carne, any food with sauces and salads for instance. The fear is that the individual does not know for sure what is in these foods. This goes for specific ingredients and likely more importantly the calorie content of these ingredients.

Distracting Behaviors

Distracting behaviors help some to divert attention from eating. As mentioned elsewhere, sucking on sugarless candy or chewing gum can distract someone from the act of eating.

Being Busy

Any task that occupies someone's attention other than eating may be employed. Watching television, searching the internet, texting, talking on the phone, studying, going for a walk and endless other behaviors are possible.

Drugs and Alcohol

Intoxication is a form of distraction. It can take one's mind off of wanting to eat over a prolonged period of time. Individuals can remain inebriated for hours or even days. Some drugs suppress appetite.

Aversion Behaviors

Aversion behaviors are those that, by observing or doing, are perceived as disgusting, repulsive or overpowering. Examples are cleaning a litter box or a dirty toilet, changing a diaper or, as personal caregivers would do, clean someone who has soiled themselves. Cleaning up one's vomit strewn around the toilet or diarrheal stool as a result of laxative abuse, are other examples. Sniffing solvents such as turpentine, gasoline as well as cleaning solvents including ammonia can be overwhelming and inhibit urges to eat.

Some find watching and listening to others eat, eating in front of a mirror or observing obese individuals repugnant.

Avoiding Behaviors

Some avoid any temptation to engage in eating including bingeing. They avoid restaurants, grocery stores, as well as eating with family and friends. Places that trigger binge eating such as the bedroom, kitchen, or car may be avoided. Medical and dietitian appointments may be avoided as this is where they will be expected to improve their nutrition as well as to stop bingeing, vomiting, over-exercising, or any other eating disorder behavior they are engaged in.

Reference

1. Kirkpatrick JR. Taking a Detailed Eating Disorder History: A Comprehensive Guide for Clinicians. *Routledge*. 2019.

Index